Jan 11-23 92

# Female and Male Climacteric

# Female and Male Climacteric

## Current Opinion 1978

Edited by P. A. van Keep,
D. M. Serr and R. B. Greenblatt

The Workshop Moderators' Reports presented at the
Second International Congress on the Menopause
held in Jerusalem, June 1978, under the auspices of
The American Geriatrics Society

University Park Press
Baltimore

Published in USA and Canada by
University Park Press
233 East Redwood Street
Baltimore, Maryland 21202

Published in UK by
MTP Press Limited
Falcon House
Lancaster, England

ISBN: 0-8391-1362-5
LCC: 78-20537

Printed in Great Britain

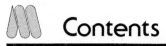 Contents

CONTENTS

# Preface

The decision taken during the First International Congress on the Menopause in June 1976 to repeat the exercise 2 years later turned out to be a good one.

In the last few years much work has been done on the subject of the menopause. It is, of course, a subject of many facets, but of particular importance recently has been the work done as a result of the reports appearing in 1975 and 1976 alleging an increase in the incidence of endometrial carcinoma in women who had used oestrogens, and of other effects, some beneficial others deleterious, reportedly seen when oestrogens were administered. 1978 seemed the right time to re-assess the situation, and the Second International Congress on the Menopause provided a good platform.

The congress was held in Jerusalem in June 1978. It took the form of a series of 12 workshops, each of which, within a prescribed framework, was planned and presided over by a moderator experienced in that particular field. The 12 moderators were free to organize their sessions in whichever way they wished, and to invite whoever they wished to present papers and to join in the discussions. In addition the workshops were open to anyone who wished to attend.

Several of the workshops were held simultaneously so it was not possible for the participants to attend all of them. On the last afternoon, however, all participants joined together to hear the moderators summarize what had been said in the workshops they had chaired, and it is these summaries which are reproduced in this book.

This format, of course, does not lead to a clear consensus of opinion. Indeed, as will be seen in the following pages, the opinions expressed in one workshop were sometimes contradictory to those expressed in another. When this occurs it is clear that more research is needed in order to clarify the matter.

The theme of the congress was 'The Female and Male Climacteric' but only one workshop dealt with the male climacteric. The opinion of the participants of this workshop was that the male climacteric as such probably does not exist, but it is the opinion of many that far more research is needed in this connection.

A number of papers read during the workshop meetings and presented during the free communications sessions have been submitted to *Maturitas* and will appear in that journal in due course.

We, the editors, are extremely grateful to the workshop moderators, all of whom worked hard to make the congress a success, and who supplied the reports which form this book. We are also grateful to Pamela Freebody who assisted with the editing task.

Our thanks are also due, and are hereby extended, to the Honorary President of the Congress, Professor Michel Albeaux-Fernet, upon whose instigation the first, and so second, congress in this series was held. Professor Menashe Ben-David, Professor Dan Hertz, Professor Bruno Lunenfeld, Dr Benjamin Maoz, and Professor Jacob Menczel joined Pieter van Keep as members of the programme committee and it is largely the enthusiasm and combined efforts of this group that resulted in the gathering together of such an interesting group of people. Finally, our thanks are due to all those, the un-named as well as the named, who attended this congress, and who, through their presence, showed the extent to which the subject of the menopause is gaining importance in the eyes of scientists of many different disciplines.

P. A. van Keep, *International Programme Co-ordinator*
D. M. Serr, *Secretary General*
R. B. Greenblatt, *Chairman*

# List of contributing participants

*Included in this list are the names and addresses of the congress officials, the workshop moderators, the participants specifically invited to contribute to the workshops, and the first-named authors of the papers presented in the free communication sessions, a list of which begins on page 140. It should be noted that, whilst most of these free communications were presented by the first-named authors, some were not; the first-named authors are given here in order that a point of contact may be established.*

**T. ABE**
Department of Obstetrics and
    Gynecology,
Tohoku University School of
    Medicine,
1–1 Seiryo-machi,
Sendai 980, Japan

**M. F. AKSU**
Department of Endocrinology,
Medical College of Georgia,
Augusta, Georgia, USA

**S. ANDERMAN**
Department of Obstetrics and
    Gynecology,
Hillel Jaffa Memorial Hospital,
Hadera, Israel

**P. ASCHHEIM**
Unité de Recherches
    Gérontologiques,
U. 118, 29 rue Wilhem,
75016 Paris, France

**M. ASSAEL**
Kaplan Hospital,
Rehovot, Israel

**C. BABUNA**
Department of Obstetrics and
    Gynecology,
Istanbul University,
Istanbul, Turkey

**S. BALLINGER**
Department of Behavioural Sciences
    in Medicine,
University of Sydney,
Sydney, NSW, Australia

**M. L. BATRINOS**
Department of Experimental
    Pharmacology of the University
    of Athens,
'Vassileus Pavlos' Hospital,
Athens, Greece

**M. BEN-DAVID**
Department of Pharmacology,
The Hebrew University,
Hadassah Medical School,
PO Box 1172,
Jerusalem, Israel

**C. BENGTSSON**
University of Gothenburg,
Department of Medicine II,
Sahlgrenska Sjukhuset,
Gothenburg SV, Sweden

**O. BENKERT**
Psychiatrische Klinik der
  Universität München,
Nussbaumstrasse 7,
8000 Munich, West Germany

**J. BONNAR**
Trinity College Unit,
Rotunda Hospital,
Dublin, Ireland

**R. BORENSTEIN**
Medical College of Georgia,
Augusta, Georgia, USA

**S. CAMPBELL**
Department of Obstetrics and
  Gynaecology,
King's College Hospital Medical
  School,
University of London,
Denmark Hill,
London SE5 8RX, United Kingdom

**M. J. CASEY**
Department of Gynecologic
  Oncology,
The University of Connecticut
  Health Center,
Farmington, Connecticut, USA

**F. COMHAIRE**
Academisch Ziekenhuis,
135 De Pintelaan,
B 9000 Ghent, Belgium

**D. W. CRAMER**
The Menopause Clinic,
Boston Hospital for Women,
Boston, Massachusetts, USA

**J. A. DAVIES**
Department of Medicine,
Martin Wing, General Infirmary,
Leeds, United Kingdom

**L. DENNERSTEIN**
Department of Psychiatry,
University of Melbourne,
c/o PO Royal Melbourne Hospital,
Victoria 3050, Australia

**M. DHONT**
Department of Gynaecology,
Akademisch Ziekenhuis,
De Pintelaan 115,
B 9000 Ghent, Belgium

**Y. Z. DIAMANT**
Hadassah Medical Relief
  Association,
Department of Obstetrics and
  Gynecology,
Kiryat Hadassah,
Jerusalem, Israel

**F. DIENSTL**
Cardiology Intensive Care Unit,
Anichstrasse 35,
6020 Innsbruck,
Austria

**P. DOERR**
Max Planck Institute for Psychiatry,
Kraepelinstrasse 10,
8 Munich 40, West Germany

**Z. DURMUS**
Ankara Maternity Hospital,
Talatpasa Bulvari,
Cebeci, Ankara, Turkey

**N. DURST**
Geha Psychiatric Hospital,
Petah-Tiqvah, Israel

**M. EUSTRATIADES**
The Laboratories of Cytology and
  Pathology of the 1st Department
  of Obstetrics and Gynecology of
  the University of Athens,
Alexandra Hospital,
Athens, Greece

**M. P. FLINT**
Department of Anthropology,
Human Biology,
Montclair State College,
Upper Montclair,
New Jersey 070043, USA

**M. FURUHJELM**
Sabbatsbergs Kvinnoklinik,
Stockholm Va, Sweden

**R. D. GAMBRELL Jr**
903 15th Street,
Augusta,
Georgia 30901, USA

**S. GELLER**
Centre d'Exploration Fonctionnelle
et d'Etude de la Reproduction
Humaine,
Laboratoire d'Hormonologie,
21, rue Edmond-Rostand,
13006 Marseille, France

**J. A. GOLDMAN**
Department of Obstetrics-
Gynecology,
Hasharon Municipal Hospital,
Tel-Aviv University Medical School,
Petah-Tiqvah, Israel

**G. S. GORDAN**
Department of Medicine,
University of California Medical
Center,
San Francisco, California, USA

**R. B. GREENBLATT**
Medical College of Georgia,
School of Medicine,
Augusta, Georgia, USA

**A. A. HASPELS**
Universiteitskliniek voor
Gynecologie en Verloskunde,
Academisch Ziekenhuis Utrecht,
Catharijnesingel 101,
Utrecht, The Netherlands

**J. HEIDENREICH**
Frauenklinik,
Universität Dusseldorf,
Moorenstrasse 5,
4 Dusseldorf 1,
West Germany

**D. HERTZ**
Department of Psychiatry,
Hadassah Medical Center,
Jerusalem, Israel

**B. HOCHSTÄDT**
The Amran Harofe Medical
Laboratory,
Rechov Balfour 3,
Haifa, Israel

**A. HOLTE**
Institute for Psychology,
University of Oslo,
PO Box 1094,
Blindern, Oslo 3, Norway

**J. HUSTIN**
Institut de Morphologie
Pathologique,
B 6270 Loverval, Belgium

**H. S. JACOBS**
Obstetric Unit,
St Mary's Hospital,
Paddington,
London, United Kingdom

**H. JACOBSON**
Albany Medical College,
Albany, New York, USA

**L. B. JASZMANN**
Department of Obstetrics and
Gynecology,
Regional Protestant Hospital,
6720 GA-Bennekom,
The Netherlands

**H. JICK**
Boston Collaborative Drug
Surveillance Program,
400 Totten Pond Road,
Waltham, Massachusetts, USA

**S. J. JOEL-COHEN**
Department of Obstetrics and
Gynecology,
The Beilinson Medical Center,
Tel-Aviv University Medical School,
Petah-Tiqvah, Israel

**P. W. JUNGBLUT**
Max Planck Institute,
PO Box 1009,
Wilhelmshaven, West Germany

**D. KASKARELIS**
Maternity Hospital 'Alexandra',
Vas. Sophias Avenue and
   K. Lourou Street,
Athens, Greece

**A. M. KAYE**
Department of Hormone Research,
The Weizmann Institute of Science,
Rehovoth, Israel

**P. A. van KEEP**
International Health Foundation,
8, avenue Don Bosco,
1150 Brussels, Belgium

**R. J. B. KING**
Imperial Cancer Research Fund,
Lincoln's Inn Fields,
London, United Kingdom

**E. S. KOHANE**
Mental Health Clinic,
Rambam University Hospital and
   A. Khouski School of Medicine,
Haifa, Israel

**H. KOPERA**
Institute of Experimental and
   Clinical Pharmacology,
University of Graz,
Universitätsplatz 4/1,
8010 Graz, Austria

**F. LABRIE**
Groupe du Conseil de Recherches
   Médicales en Endocrinologie
   Moléculaire,
Centre Hospitalier de l'Université
   Laval,
2705 Boulevard Laurier,
Quebec GIV 4 G2, Canada

**U. LACHNIT-FIXON**
Schering AG,
Postfach 65.0311,
Mullerstrasse 170,
1 Berlin 65, West Germany

**E. LANDAU**
Rechov Hess, 8,
Tel-Aviv, Israel

**U. LARSSON-COHN**
Department of Obstetrics and
   Gynecology,
University Hospital,
Linköping, Sweden

**C. LAURITZEN**
Universität Ulm,
Frauenklinik,
Prittwitzstrasse 43,
79 Ulm, West Germany

**P. E. LEBECH**
Department of Obstetrics and
   Gynaecology,
Frederiksberg Hospital,
2000 Copenhagen,
Denmark

**H. M. LEMON**
Section of Oncology,
Department of Internal Medicine,
University of Nebraska Medical
   Center,
42nd Street and Dewey Avenue,
Omaha, Nebraska, USA

**O. LINDQUIST**
Departments of Medicine and
   Obstetrics and Gynecology,
University of Gothenburg,
Gothenburg, Sweden

**R. LINDSAY**
Western Infirmary,
Glasgow, United Kingdom

**P. F. A. van LOOK**
Department of Obstetrics and
  Gynecology,
Leiden University Hospital,
Leiden, The Netherlands

**B. LUNENFELD**
Department of Endocrinology,
Chaim Sheba Medical Center,
Tel Hashomer, Israel

**S. J. MANTALENAKIS**
First Department of Obstetrics and
  Gynecology,
University of Thessaloniki,
Al. Papanastasiou 50,
Thessaloniki, Greece

**B. MAOZ**
Geha Psychiatric Hospital,
Kupat Holim,
PO Box 72,
Petah-Tiqvah, Israel

**D. McKAY HART**
Stobhill General Hospital,
Glasgow, United Kingdom

**J. MENCZEL**
Ministry of Health,
Jerusalem, Israel

**J. MENCZER**
Department of Obstetrics and
  Gynecology,
Chaim Sheba Medical Center,
Tel Hashomer, Israel

**H. MUSAPH**
Academisch Ziekenhuis Utrecht,
Afdeling Sexuologie,
Catharijnesingel 101,
3500 CG Utrecht, The Netherlands

**T. NENCIONI**
Seconda Clinica Ostetrico-
  Ginecologica dell'Università
  degli Studi di Milano,
Via Commenda 12,
20122 Milan, Italy

**J. NEVINNY-STICKEL**
Frauenklinik und Poliklinik
  Charlottenburg,
Freie Universität Berlin,
FB 3, WE 14, Pulsstrasse 4–14,
1000 Berlin 19, West Germany

**E. NIESCHLAG**
Abt. Experimentelle Endokrinologie,
Universitäts-Frauenklinik,
Westring 11,
4400 Munich, West Germany

**M. NOTELOVITZ**
Department of Obstetrics and
  Gynecology,
The University of Florida College
  of Medicine,
Box J-294, JHMHC,
Gainesville, Florida, USA

**M. OETTINGER**
Reproductive Biology Unit,
Rothschild University Hospital,
Haifa, Israel

**D. H. ORAM**
Department of Obstetrics and
  Gynecology,
University of Natal Medical School,
King Edward VII Hospital,
Durban, South Africa

**M. E. L. PATERSON**
Department of Obstetrics and
  Gynaecology,
University of Birmingham,
Birmingham, United Kingdom

**H. PETERS**
The Finsen Laboratory,
Finsen Institute,
Strandboulevarden 49,
Copenhagen 2100,
Denmark

**G. A. PUCA**
Istituto Patologia Generale I
  Facolta Medicina,
S. Andreadame 2,
Naples, Italy

**R. RUBENS**
Academisch Ziekenhuis,
135 De Pintelaan,
9000 Ghent, Belgium

**T. SALMI**
Department of Obstetrics and
Gynecology,
Turku University Hospital,
Turku, Finland

**G. SAMSIOE**
University of Gothenburg,
Sahlgrenska Sjukhuset,
Gothenburg SV, Sweden

**A. SCHACHTER**
Gynecologic Cytology and
Colposcopy Unit,
Beilinson Medical Center,
Petah-Tiqvah, Israel

**A. M. C. M. SCHELLEN**
Gynecological Department,
R.C. Hospital,
Sittard, The Netherlands

**J. G. SCHENKER**
Hadassah Medical Relief
Association,
Department of Obstetrics and
Gynecology,
Kirvat Hadassah,
Jerusalem, Israel

**H. SCHMIDT**
Klinik für Diagnostik,
Aukamallee 33,
Postfach 2149,
Wiesbaden, West Germany

**H. SCHNEIDER**
Evangelisches Krankenhaus,
Waldstrasse 73,
Bad Godesberg 1,
5300 Bonn, West Germany

**H. P. G. SCHNEIDER**
Universitäts-Fraùenklinik,
Westring 11,
Munich, West Germany

**L. SCHUBERT**
Department of Obstetrics and
Gynecology,
University of Milano,
Via Commenda 12,
Milan, Italy

**U. SCHWARTZ**
Division of Gynecologic
Endocrinology,
Sterility and Family Planning,
Department of Obstetrics and
Gynecology,
Klinikum Steglitz,
Free University of Berlin,
Berlin, West Germany

**M. SERIO**
Endocrinology Unit,
University of Florence,
Florence, Italy

**D. M. SERR**
Department of Obstetrics and
Gynecology,
Chaim Sheba Medical Center,
Tel Hashomer, Israel

**E. van SEUMEREN**
Gynecology Ward,
University Hospital,
Catharijnesingel 101,
Utrecht, The Netherlands

**L. SEVERNE**
International Health Foundation,
43 rue de Namur/Boîte n° 5,
1000 Brussels, Belgium

**Y. SHANAN**
Department of Psychiatry,
Hadassah Medical Center,
Jersualem, Israel

**D. R. SHANKLIN**
Department of Obstetrics/
Gynecology and Pathology,
University of Chicago,
Chicago, USA

**R. L. SITRUK-WARE**
Service d'Endocrinologie et de
  Gynécologie Médicale –
  Assistance Publique,
Hôpitaux de Paris – Hôpital Necker,
149 rue de Sèvres,
75730 Paris Cédex 15, France

**H. SKÖLDEFORS**
Sabbatsbergs Kvinnoklinik,
Stockholm Va, Sweden

**J. R. STRECKER**
Universitätsfrauenklinik,
Prittwitzstrasse 43,
Ulm, West Germany

**J. W. W. STUDD**
King's College Hospital,
Denmark Hill,
London SE5 9RS,
United Kingdom

**D. W. STURDEE**
Department of Gynaecology,
Walsgrave Hospital,
Coventry, United Kingdom

**G. B. TALBERT**
Department of Anatomy and Cell
  Biology,
Downstate Medical Center,
450 Clarkson Street,
Brooklyn, New York, USA

**J. H. H. THIJSSEN**
Academisch Ziekenhuis Utrecht,
Universiteitskliniek voor Inwendige
  Geneeskunde – Klinische
  Endocrinologie,
Catharijnesingel 101,
Utrecht, The Netherlands

**M. H. THOM**
Dulwich Hospital,
London SE22, United Kingdom

**J. L. TOY**
University Department of Medicine,
General Infirmary,
Leeds LS1 3EX, United Kingdom

**W. H. UTIAN**
Case Western Reserve University,
University Circle,
Cleveland, Ohio, USA

**M. I. WHITEHEAD**
Department of Obstetrics and
  Gynaecology,
King's College Hospital Medical
  School,
Denmark Hill,
London SE5 8RX, United Kingdom

**M. A. H. M. WIEGERINCK**
Department of Obstetrics and
  Gynecology,
University Hospital,
Catharijnesingel 101,
Utrecht, The Netherlands

**J. WILBUSH**
Grimshaw Medical Clinic,
PO Box 209,
Grimshaw, Alberta TOH 1WO,
Canada

**V. ZARAGOZÀ ORTS**
Servicio de Ginecologia,
Hospital Provincial,
Valencia, Spain

## Note

*Names appearing in parentheses and followed by a year indicate that the preceding statement has been published elsewhere. Relevant details will be found in the list of references at the end of each chapter.*

*A name unaccompanied by a year indicates that the preceding statement or viewpoint was expressed by that person in the course of the congress.*

**1** Workshop report

# Sociology and anthropology of the menopause

Moderator: M. P. Flint
Montclair State College, Upper Montclair, New Jersey, USA

*Participants invited to present their views at this
workshop included:*

*A. Holte (Norway)*
*P. A. van Keep (Belgium)*
*B. Maoz (Israel)*
*H. Musaph (The Netherlands)*
*H. Schneider (West Germany)*
*L. Severne (Belgium)*
*J. Wilbush (Canada)*

## INTRODUCTION

There are two aspects of the menopause which researchers have studied – the somatic or biological and the environmental, which is either organic or cultural. This cultural imposition is important, as it influences two areas of menopause research which have traditionally been investigated by physicians and social and behavioural scientists – the age at which this phenomenon occurs and the types and severity of symptoms which are ascribed to this event. To understand and treat a menopausal woman without understanding the cultural *Gestalt* which has influenced her all the years of her life up to this time, is to ignore what may be the most important determinants of how a woman responds to the menopause both physically

1

and behaviourally. As Levine and Dougherty have noted, 'Only when the whole woman is considered in her day to day living can the old combination of mental, physical and social systems that appear at menopause be understood' (Levine and Dougherty, 1952).

## AGE AT MENOPAUSE

Factors that affect age at menopause have been summarized as well as suggested as topics for future research by Fling (Fling, 1976). In this workshop the factors that might influence age at menopause were briefly discussed (van Keep). In a study undertaken by the International Health Foundation in 1977 of over 6000 Dutch women in Ede, which was the same population studied by Jaszmann some 10 years earlier (Jaszmann et al., 1969), it was hoped that a secular trend in age at menopause would be shown between these 10-year cohort groups; however, it was not, with both the 1967 and 1977 groups having a median age of menopause at 51.4 years, as determined by the probit method of analysis. This study does indicate, though, that cohort or generational studies of 20 years, rather than 10 years, may be more appropriate to test this secular trend.

The IHF did find cultural factors which correlated with an earlier or later mean age at menopause among those women of this Ede population who were post-menopausal. Factors found to be of importance – in the sense that they are associated with an earlier menopause – are:

- working outside of the home (a factor strongly related to marital status, since it was mainly single women who did so);
- smoking;
- having smoked in the past;
- height under 1.55 m;
- body weight under 60 kg.

The study indicates that a pregnancy after the age of 40 is correlated with a later menopause but the data are non-conclusive. The same can be said of prolonged oral contraceptive use, but the group of women who had used the pill for a considerable time and who were now post-menopausal is too small to allow for a firm conclusion to be made on this point (Brand and Lehert, 1978). Certainly, this IHF study points out the continued need for cross-cultural research of those factors which may universally influence the age at which this reproductive landmark occurs.

2

## HISTORICAL PERSPECTIVE ON MENOPAUSAL SYMPTOMATOLOGY

A unique approach to the study of menopausal symptomatologies is that suggested by Wilbush who has done an exhaustive search on the historical 'birth of the menopause syndrome' in France. He attributes the term, *La Ménespausie*, to Gardanne who in the early 1800s wrote the first text entirely devoted to disturbances at the female climacteric (Gardanne, 1816). Wilbush suggests that culture has historically conditioned climacteric symptomatology. He points out that in ancient times these were not referred to, although the classical literature of Rome, Byzantium and post-Renaissance Europe contains numerous references to age at menopause, as well as remedies for menochesis, 'retention of the menses', but little to disturbances at this time. For example, in France it is suggested that the symptomatologies of ladies of the upper classes were mainly due to the reification of social stresses after the revolution. Promiscuity, venereal disease, and a rising incidence of cancer, as well as increased use of emmenagogues and other medications to counteract the cessation of menstruation, and, with this, the ageing process, are believed to have added a considerable element of physical debility to the great mental strain women were subject to at this historical period. Medical practices in post-revolutionary France, by then having switched for women from *sage-femmes* to physicians, allowed the presentation for the first time of these symptoms, which made the doctors aware of the strain which the 'change of life' imposed on some women. Wilbush's study of the French literature and the genesis of menopausal symptomatology there suggests the need for more library research in other countries which have early medical literature, particularly in Europe.

## CULTURAL AND SOCIAL INFLUENCES ON MENOPAUSAL SYMPTOMATOLOGY

### Culture and cognition

Another approach to the study of menopausal symptoms was offered by Holte who suggests that rather than relate causality of symptomatology to hormonal changes occurring in women belonging to high-frequency groups, one must also look at the social and cognitive circumstances under which physiological changes are occurring in women at this time of life. He feels that women of high-frequency groups are in a situation similar to that of test subjects in a Schachter and Singer social–psychological experiment on the cognitive, social and physiological determinants of emotional states (Schachter and Singer, 1962). The high-frequency groups share a common frame of interpretation of the menopause as a function of their specific sex-role attitudes. Culture then presents a ready-made frame of interpretation which determines what to feel when physiological changes of the climacteric period arrive, for these women. The cultural framework determines whether the physiologically produced sensations will be manifest as psychosomatic and psychosocial problems of the menopause or not. Further, the knowledge of the sex-role patterns of the high-frequency groups may then be related to establishing theories and noting experiences from clinical psychology about family interaction. Important determinants of the psychosomatic and especially psychosocial problems of the climacteric women in high-frequency groups can also be found in the life situations of their husbands of corresponding ages. Holte's research suggests that family studies of peri-menopausal women are much needed and are an area of research little studied till now.

## Work and symptomatology

Schneider presented a study of 2232 women in West Germany who were either agricultural workers or who had independent professions at the time of the climacteric. One of the strong points of this study is the relationship of work to menopausal symptomatologies and health generally. It was found that adequate physical adaptation to work is of great importance, as is attitude about work. Women with independent positions, for example, feel that they 'cannot afford to be ill'. With this attitude some symptoms of the menopause are then repressed or do not develop in this group, while agricultural workers also reported less symptoms of menopause and illness generally.

Besides this attitude about the work, socio-psychological factors studied among agricultural women, specifically, come into play. Women of this group feel healthier if they are unburdened in the household, having the assistance of other family members. A patri-archial family structure is also felt to influence the repression of any symptoms (of the menopause or other illness). Finally, motivation for working and the extent to which a woman can really practise her job are important influences on symptomalogy for all women, in both these groups. If a woman is well motivated for her profession, if she can practise her work, and if she is unburdened with house-work, she is more likely to be healthy during the climacteric age and to suffer few symptoms. Also, if she has never had a job (or had one for only a short time) and has had the traditional role of mother and wife, she will remain healthy with few, if any, symptoms. If, however, she is forced to stay at home with children, when she would prefer to go out to work, her symptoms will be greater.

A positive correlation between the matrimonial situation and climacteric symptoms of these women is also seen (Prill, 1969). Women with severe symptoms are generally more friendless and refuse social contacts, as well as experiencing more stresses in the home. This study suggests that if duties at home do not cause excessive stress, part-time workers show less depressive reactions, less functional heart diseases and fewer symptoms of the climacteric, than women who are full-time housewives. Some limited occupation other than housework is felt to have a favourable effect on the climacteric period.

Another paper which also stresses the role of work and the role of the housewife in relation to climacteric symptoms was that pre-sented by Severne. She reviewed the findings of a 1974 study by the International Health Foundation of 922 Belgian women in the pre-, peri- and post-menopausal stages of life and reported on the influ-ence of their roles as women, and their socio-economic status on attitudes, behaviour and symptomatology. The findings of this study first refute the misconception that menopause is a pseudo-ailment of the privileged classes, although women who have higher material and educational standards and who live in more stimulating en-vironments, with more resources and possible choices in life, are found to be less prone to the difficulties of the climacteric. While work is generally considered to have a favourable influence on menopausal women, this too is found to be socially differentiated. For the upper socio-economic group of women, working outside the home is practically always favourable; however, this is not found among women of the lower socio-economic group. Having a job for this latter group brings stress and tension during the peri-meno-pause. Among women in both classes, however, having a job during the post-menopause is found to be a stabilizing factor.

It is also noted in this study that housewives of both classes are more vulnerable than women who work outside of the house to

5

climacteric complaints. However, this too is socially differentiated. Housewives of the lower socio-economic group report more symptoms and complaints than those of the upper socio-economic group. All in all though, housewives generally appear to be at a disadvantage, particularly in the post-menopause. They suffer more severely and more frequently from the long-lasting effects of the climacteric, both somatically and psychologically. Severne suggests, much as does Schneider, that for the housewife, a greater involvement in all sectors of life, outside of the home would have decided advantages during the peri- and post-menopausal stages of life.

Maoz, however, cautioned against the stereotypical advice of physicians to menopausal women 'to go out and get a job'. In a study of five ethnic groups of women who had migrated into Israel, a low incidence of climacteric complaints was found among European Jews, and Arabs in the peri- and post-menopause, where their work load was unchanged or was somewhat more than before this time period (Maoz *et al.*, 1978). Persian Jews, on the other hand, showed a sharp contrast to this – those who had never worked outside of the home suffered less than any other group of women at all stages of the menopause. This difference cannot be explained by socio-economic differences among the five groups, but rather by a multiplicity of factors including physical health, marital relationships, and general stability.

## SEXUALITY AND CLIMACTERIC COMPLAINTS

Musaph briefly described the menopause as triggering problems, both psychological and somatic, at this time of life. It has been suggested that, for the climacteric woman, coital frequency is reduced (Kinsey *et al.*, 1953; Masters and Johnson, 1970), but the inter-relationship of frequency of sexual relations and of climacteric complaints has yet to be fully studied cross-culturally. Hällström has done some work on this topic in Sweden (Hällström, 1977), but his results to date do not suggest strong correlations between these two factors.

## CONCLUSIONS

As can be seen by the varied approaches to the study of the climacteric, the cultural aspect, as well as the biological one, is quite significant. As such, there are a multitude of factors waiting to be investigated cross-culturally. This workshop leads one to suggest but a few of these: (1) secular trend studies every generation or 20 years for age at menopause, (2) the effects of smoking, oral contraceptive pill, height, and weight on age at menopause, (3) library research for the earliest references of menopause and climacteric complaints and treatment in ancient civilizations, classical literature, and historical literature (particularly in Europe for this last group), (4) perception and cognition of what the menopause and climacteric complaints are about, (5) family interactions during the climacteric phase of life, (6) the role of work, both within and outside the home on age at menopause and its symptoms or complaints, and (7) the relationship of sexual behaviour to the climacteric syndrome.

Finally, it can be suggested that most cultural studies of the menopause to date are actually national studies. What is needed in future research is to show how a specific culture or sub-culture (ethnic group) views the menopause, has attitudes, beliefs, and values about this time of life that are unique to a specific population, and in what ways this influences both men and women around the time of the menopause. With adequate data from these types of studies, we may then proceed to do cross-cultural comparisons among varied populations.

## References

Brand, P. C. and Lehert, P. (1978). A new way of looking at environmental variables that may affect the age at menopause. *Maturitas*, **1**, 121

Flint, M. (1976). Cross-cultural factors that affect age of menopause. In: *Consensus on Menopause Research* (P. A. van Keep, R. B. Greenblatt and M. Albeaux-Fernet, eds.), pp. 73–83. (Lancaster: MTP Press)

Gardanne, C. P. L. (1816). Avis aux femmes qui entrent dans l'age critique. (Paris)

Hällström, T. (1977). Sexuality in the climacteric. *Clin. Obstet. Gynecol.*, **4**, 227

Jaszmann, L., Lith, N. D. van and Zaat, J. C. A. (1969). The perimenopausal symptoms: The statistical analysis of a survey. *Med. Gynaecol. Sociol.*, **4**, 268

Kinsey, A. C., Pomeroy, W. B., Martin, C. E. and Gebhard, P. H. (1953). *Sexual Behaviour in the Human Female*. (Philadelphia: W. B. Saunders)

Levine, L. and Dougherty, B. (1952). *The Menopause*. (New York: Random House)

Maoz, B., Antonovsky, A., Apter, A., Datan, N., Hochberg, J. and Salomon, Y. (1978). The effect of outside work on the menopausal woman. *Maturitas*, **1**, 43

Masters, W. H. and Johnson, V. E. (1970). *Human Sexual Inadequacy*. (Boston: Little, Brown)

Prill, H. J. (1969). Symptome durch die Arbeitsbelastung der Frau 'in der kritischen Mitte'. In: *Gesundheit, Arbeit und Produktivität*. Bundesausschuss für gesundheitliche Volksbelehrung e.V.

Schachter, S. and Singer, J. (1962). Cognitive, social and physiological determinants of emotional state. *Psychol. Rev.*, **69**, 379

# Psychology of the menopause

## Moderator: B. Maoz

## Secretary: N. Durst

Geha Psychiatric Hospital, The Beilinson Medical Centre, Tel-Aviv University Medical School, Tel-Aviv, Israel

*Participants invited to present their views at this workshop included:*

*M. Assael (Israel)*
*L. Dennerstein (Australia)*
*N. Durst (Israel)*
*M. P. Flint (USA)*
*A. A. Haspels (The Netherlands)*
*D. Hertz (Israel)*
*L. B. Jaszmann (The Netherlands)*
*E. Landau (Israel)*
*H. Musaph (The Netherlands)*
*E. van Seumeren (The Netherlands)*
*Y. Shanan (Israel)*

The discussions in this workshop concerned three main topics:

(1) Psychological aspects of the normal development of climacteric women.

(2) Psychopathology of the climacterium.

(3) Some aspects of patient management and therapy, in particular the effects of oestrogen therapy on psychological well-being and functioning.

## PSYCHOLOGICAL ASPECTS

The stage of life known as the climacteric phase is a normal transitional stage (Shanan). During the last century, menarche has started at a younger age and, as a consequence, the fertile period has become longer. But at the same time the whole life expectancy has risen much more and thus the fertile period in a woman's life has become relatively shorter. In a study of a normal population Shanan found that during a transitional stage many forms of minor suffering may arise among men as well as among women. He investigated samples in Israel composed of three groups – one-third kibbutz members, one-third people from development communities (new immigrants), and one-third from larger towns. He found no real differences between the sexes or the three populations regarding their reaction to minor suffering. This he concluded from a longitudinal study of 500 people (male and female) aged between 45 and 65 observed from 1967 until the present time. Careful longitudinal biological and psychological investigations are important and certainly give more reliable information than cross-sectional studies. In this study it was found that the differences within an age group were mostly related to life experiences. These experiences were largely connected to specific historical events such as the economic recession of the 1920s and World War II of the 1940s through which this particular age group passed. Alongside such events, were more personal experiences such as migration, confinement in a concentration camp, malnutrition, long-term drug or medication use, all of which had a strong influence on the ability to cope in times of stress, such as the climacteric. Over a long period of time, there was little change in a person's basic coping pattern or in his mental health. No sex stereotypes were found, but generally women held up better than their ageing male counterparts (Shanan).

The interaction between wife and husband during the climacteric was discussed. Gynaecologists often deal with women whose real problem is the much more severe crisis occurring in the husband, particularly in the Western European middle class where a man's career is most important to him at this age. Whilst wishing to continue the climb up the social ladder, the middle-aged man finds his physiological functioning decreasing and his body demanding more rest. The result is a discongruity which may lead to disease, such as coronary heart disease. It is important, therefore, to pay attention to the balance existing in the relationship between the husband and the wife, both of whom may be regarded as being 'climacteric' (Jaszmann) (Jaszmann, 1978).

Each sub-culture is unique in its attitude towards menopause, and the cultural and ethnic backgrounds have their implications in the attitude of the woman towards the menopause (Flint, 1975). Two different ethnic groups were studied, one of Cuban immigrants and the other of American-born Jewish women. Among the salient differences between the two groups was the fact that the Cubans were much more reserved than the Jews concerning sex, and that they experienced menopause in a much more negative fashion than did their Jewish counterparts. It was found that only by using a female Cuban immigrant interviewer (a co-investigator in this project) could this intimate subject be studied (Flint).

The importance of the anticipation of old age and dying for the perception of menopause was introduced (Landau) (Landau and Maoz, 1978). The importance of previous self-actualization during the three earlier stages of female development: girlhood, woman-hood and motherhood was underlined. Women who had undergone these three stages in a creative manner are able to adapt and be flexible during the climacteric and in old age. Early education towards creativity is, therefore, very important. Self-actualization is easier for a woman living in a traditional society, because her social role and status are clearly defined. Women from more modern societies must find new areas of self-actualization after the role of motherhood. A study carried out in a home for the aged has shown that even old people are capable of discovering creative and original alternatives if they have been accustomed to doing so in their younger days. This ability enables them to be content in the last third of their lives without clinging to old habits, and they are thus able to cope better with the problem of death (Landau).

## PSYCHOPATHOLOGICAL ASPECTS

Some fundamental questions were raised: (a) does a special noso-logical psychopathological entity, related to the climacteric, exist? and (b) can a certain pre-morbid personality, which tends to develop this syndrome during the climacteric, be found? The participants in this workshop were divided in their answers to these two questions. The view was expressed that the menopause only shapes the 'patho-plastic' symptomatology, but that it should not be regarded as an aetiological 'pathogenic' factor. Peri-menopausal women often 'act' their complaints according to what their families expect of them, and to their 'social learning', i.e. what they remember of the experience of their own mothers. The existence of hysterical features resulting in secondary gains may be presumed (Musaph). The clinical features are a result of the pre-existent problems rooted in childhood and the expectation pattern in certain folklore (cultures) regarding disease in general and menopause in particular. A specific nosological entity may not exist, but the personality structure and its experience in early life may be of paramount importance.

Contrasting conservative views were also put forward. The traditional outlook of the Kraepelin psychiatry was presented (Kraepelin, 1907), and the existence of a special nosologic entity called 'involutional melancholia' was insisted upon (Assael). This melancholia differs from endogenous and reactive depression in the following respects:

(a)  no former affective illness;
(b)  longer duration of the disease (7–9 months);
(c)  characteristic phenomenology (with hysterical traits);
(d)  no past manic phase;
(e)  agitated behaviour;
(f)  no diurnal fluctuation.

A specific pre-morbid personality is presumed which is anal-sadistic and domineering. The climacteric involutional depression is a continuation into the period of menopause of the patient's pre-climacteric condition. The psychological conflicts of the middle-aged woman, including the cessation of menstruation, are factors which trigger off the involutional melancholia (Assael). This view met with little support; in modern literature, the so-called involutional melancholia is regarded rather as a sub-type of the unipolar (endogenous) depression (Rosenthal, 1974). The existence of a specific circumscribed pre-morbid personality structure which tends to break down easily during the climacteric phase and which may consequently develop the above-mentioned psychosis, was also rejected by most participants.

12

The modern psychosomatic approach was put forward and strongly supported. The symptomatology of the climacteric is seen as a *resultante* of various factors: biological (hormonal), psychic, and social. It is an interaction between aspects of the ageing process and the hormonal change, which may, in certain personality types, cause a temporary dysfunction (crisis). The person must be seen as a whole: that is, as an individual and as a member of her family, of society, and, of her culture.

There are influences from the past, but of no less importance are the situational stresses of life today and the anticipation of old age (Hertz). The content of the intra-psychic experiences, which change during this period of life, is important, and has been demonstrated by a study into the substance of day-dreaming by climacteric women receiving psychotherapeutic treatment (Hertz, 1976).

The fundamental question of whether or not one is justified in speaking about the existence of the climacteric syndrome was raised (Wilbush). Findings and basic research into the historical development of this syndrome (see Workshop 1 on the sociology and anthropology of the menopause) strongly suggest that the diagnosis is entirely dependent on the bias of the examining, usually male, physician.

In summarizing this section, it may be said that the participants agreed that the possible crisis during the climacteric has its roots in the following multicausal factors:

(a) psycho-sexual development starting in early childhood and resulting in a particular, individual personality pattern;

(b) certain biological stresses during the climacteric phase, such as the hormonal changes and cessation of menstruation and fertility, and the general health situation;

(c) psychological stresses, partly as an aspect of the anticipation of old age and death by the woman and her family;

(d) environmental, social, and cultural factors which shape the behaviour and outlook of the woman in crises. These bio-psycho-social factors are strongly interrelated with each other.

Only one participant described a specific psychotic disease of the climacteric woman, but even he tried to reach a synthesis between this classic viewpoint and the above-mentioned psychosomatic, holistic approach as set out by Lipowski (Assael) (Lipowski, 1976).

## PATIENT MANAGEMENT AND THERAPY

It is, of course, important to realize that not every complaint described by a patient at the time of the menopause is necessarily due to the climacteric. Complaints may be expressions of pre-existing conflicts, or may occur around the time of the menopause by sheer coincidence. The experience gained at the Academic Hospital of Utrecht (The Netherlands), which has a special menopause clinic, is illustrative, in this connection. It has been found that women between 45 and 55 years of age are under-represented in the out-patient clinic of the Department of Internal Medicine, suggesting that symptoms and complaints of women in this age group are often attributed to the climacteric rather than to problems in the field of internal medicine. For this reason it was decided that the staff of the menopause clinic should be multidisciplinary and that, in addition to being given a gynaecological examination, every patient reporting to the clinic should have a complete general medical check-up. When the results of these examinations and of the laboratory and X-ray findings are known these are discussed with the patient in an open non-authoritative way. The therapy too, is a matter of joint discussion and decision. In this rather special group of patients, often problem cases referred by general practitioners, the complaints are frequently non-climacteric in origin. About 25% of all new patients are referred to the social worker attached to the team. A small number of patients are seen by a psychiatrist or by other specialists. Only some of the patients need hormonal therapy. This underlines the necessity of a thorough general examination, a check-up which should include an investigation of the woman's psycho-social situation (van Seumeren, Haspels).

The fact that oestrogen therapy affects not only true climacteric symptoms but also the woman's psychological well-being, is evident from the following studies.

A double-blind, cross-over study (Dennerstein), was conducted on a group of hysterectomized and oophorectomized women who were treated with:

(a) oestrogen (ethinyl oestradiol);
(b) progestogen (norgestrel);

(c)  a combination of an oestrogen and a progestogen;
(d)  a placebo.

Positive results were found only in the group receiving oestrogen. Oestrogen therapy certainly improves the woman's general feelings and mood, and diminishes anxiety and irritability (all measured by objective methods). This result was obtained when treatment was given for at least 3 months. Fluctuations in the oestrogen level may cause transitional symptoms: for instance, when the level of oestrogen falls, the patient may suffer headaches (Dennerstein).

In another study (Durst and Maoz) post-menopausal women with a high score on an adapted Blatt Menopausal Index were treated for 1 year with conjugated oestrogens (Premarin). The menopausal symptoms, the degree of neuroticism and of functioning and participation in daily life were measured before, during and after treatment. The sample was homogenous and there were two matched control groups. A preliminary conclusion is that the mere provision of information about basic facts concerning the menopause during the first interview had important effects: a positive one by diminishing fear and anxiety (in 15% of cases), and a negative one by provoking drop-outs because of fear of 'that dangerous hormone treatment' (5%). Treatment was started with a placebo, but when symptoms increased (or remained unchanged), oestrogen therapy was initiated. One of the findings was that in 25% of the sample the placebo initially had a positive effect. After 2–3 months, however, the symptoms returned and the women had then to be given oestrogen therapy. Only two of the 80 women involved in this study completed 1 year on a placebo. Oestrogen therapy was also shown to have a very dramatic effect also on various non-somatic symptoms, viz.: depressed mood, anxiety, and hypochondriac worries. It caused the treated women to be more optimistic, and more satisfied, and increased their feelings of self-esteem; all measured by objective methods.

The best results were found in housewives without outside employment and women who had a high score in the index of symptoms. On the other hand, it was noted that in one of the control groups, those women who did not work outside the home and who were not treated with oestrogens, developed a higher degree of depression and anxiety, confirming the findings of an earlier study (Maoz et al., 1978).

15

The results of these two studies are very similar. In both studies objective scales and psychological tests were used.

## CONCLUSION

The psychological aspects of the climacteric may be affected and/or moderated (if necessary) in various ways depending on the goal/target of the therapist.

In certain selected women suffering from complaints, and in whom no contraindications exist, oestrogen substitution therapy can be used very successfully, also as a psychotonic drug. But this does not rule out the usefulness of other methods of treatment such as large-scale information and education, psychotherapy, and social guidance, as well as the use of tranquillizers and anti-depressant drugs. The therapist has to decide, according to the personality of the patient, how he wishes to interpose in this complex syndrome.

The participants in this workshop felt that, in the discussion about the problems of menopause, there is a lack of interdisciplinary communication – between somatically oriented specialists on the one hand, and psychiatrists and behavioural scientists on the other. Better communication would most certainly lead to a more integrated model of the peri-menopausal woman, and to a better interdisciplinary strategy for therapeutic programmes.

## References

Flint, M. (1975). The menopause: reward or punishment? *Psychosomatics*, **16**, 161

Hertz, D. G. (1976). Dreaming process and fantasy-life in menopausal women. Presented at the *1st International Congress on the Menopause,* June, La Grande Motte, France

Jaszmann, L. (1978). *De Middelbare leeftijd van de Man.* (Deventer: Van Loghum Slaterus)

Kraepelin, E. (1907). *Clinical Psychiatry* (A. R. Diefendorf, transl.) (New York: MacMillan)

Landau, E. and Maoz, B. (1978). Creativity and self-actualization in the aging personality. *Am. J. Psychother.*, **32**, **1**, 117

Lipowski, Z. J. (1976). Psychosomatic medicine: an overview. In: *Modern Trends in Psychosomatic Medicine – 3* (O. W. Hill, ed.), pp. 1–20. (London: Butterworths)

Maoz, B., Antonovsky, A., Apter, A., Datan, N., Hochberg, J. and Salomon, Y. (1978). The effect of outside work on the menopausal woman. *Maturitas*, **1**, 43

Rosenthal, S. R. (1974). Involutional depression. In: *American Handbook of Psychiatry*, 2nd ed. (S. Arielie, ed.), vol. 3, pp. 694–709. (New York: Basic Books)

**3** Workshop report

# The ageing ovary

## Moderator: H. Peters

The Finsen Laboratory,
Copenhagen, Denmark

*Participants invited to present their views at this
workshop included:*

*P. Aschheim (France)*
*H. S. Jacobs (United Kingdom)*
*R. Rubens (Belgium)*
*G. B. Talbert (USA)*

## INTRODUCTION

The ageing of the ovary is a gradual process which occurs during the
period that lies between full fertility and final sterility. The changes
that occur in the ovary influence the hypothalamic–pituitary unit
and their hormone production which, in turn, influence the hormone
production and functions of the ovary itself. All the oocytes a woman
will have during her lifetime are enclosed in small follicles and are
already present in the ovary at birth. A human ovary contains about
700 000 small follicles when the child is born; this number is reduced
to half by the time menarche occurs. A reduction in number
continues throughout the fertile period and only a few are left at
menopause. In addition to a progressive decrease in the number of
small follicles there occurs a distinct reduction in the number of
antral follicles in the ovaries of pre-menopausal women.

## AGEING CHANGES IN THE OVARY OF THE LABORATORY MOUSE (Introduced by G. B. Talbert)

Before the complete cessation of fertility a period of reproductive decline occurs. The decline seen in the laboratory mouse occurs at a time that is comparable in the human to the years prior to menopause; during this period pregnancies are more difficult to achieve and to maintain than earlier. This decline in reproductive capacity is not due to exhaustion of oocytes or failure of ovulation. Ageing mice ovulate as many eggs as young ones.

Several factors are responsible for this change: the uterus becomes increasingly unable to support pregnancy, and a decrease in the viability of ova becomes important. The oocyte remains in prophase throughout the resting phase of the small follicle. This prolonged stage, which may extend for up to 50 years in the human and for over a year in the mouse, may be responsible for an increase in chromosomal abnormalities in the oocyte of older women and mice, leading to abnormalities and loss of the conceptus. Delayed ovulation, occurring frequently in older individuals, may also be associated with loss of viability of ova. In addition to the ageing of the oocyte itself, a decline in the endocrine function may be a contributing factor. In ageing animals the corpora lutea of early pregnancy show some morphological changes not seen in younger individuals; however, no evidence of qualitative changes in LH binding sites in corpora lutea has been found. Furthermore, differences in progesterone levels in blood of young and ageing pregnant mice have not been seen.

## FACTORS INFLUENCING OVARIAN AGEING (Introduced by P. Aschheim)

Extrinsic and intrinsic factors influence ovarian ageing. Several changes occur in the ageing ovary: there is a marked proliferation of the surface epithelium leading to cysts and deep invaginations, which carry cells from the surface into the substance of the ovary itself; pigment-bearing phagocytes become increasingly more frequent; furthermore structures appear in the ovary, consisting of nodules and ducts, which might become very extensive with advancing age. The question arises, which of these changes are due to ageing in the pituitary and which occur primarily in the ovary, independent of the pituitary ageing? Experiments in which the pituitary was removed from young animals have shown that the ovaries of ageing, hypophysectomized animals do not show the proliferation of the surface epithelium nor the appearance of pigment bearing phagocytes. The absence of the pituitary, however, did not prevent the marked proliferation of ducts which have been suggested to be a proliferation of the rete ovarii. It was emphasized that probably none of the ageing changes in the ovary is entirely intrinsic.

## HORMONE PRODUCTION OF THE AGEING OVARY
(Introduced by R. Rubens)

Consideration was given to the questions: which hormones are still secreted by the post-menopausal ovary, and what factors influence sex hormone levels in post-menopausal women? The ovary maintains a substantial secretory function after the menopause. The levels of sex hormones in the intact post-menopausal woman are fairly low. In ovariectomized, post-menopausal women a further lowering of androgens (testosterone, dihydrotestosterone and androstenedione) is observed, while the oestrogens levels remain similar. In order to determine the contribution of the sex steroids by the adrenal, suppression (by dexamethasone) and stimulation (by ACTH) of the adrenals were used. Suppression of the adrenals caused a 60% decrease in the circulating oestrone and oestradiol levels, while stimulation doubled the levels of these oestrogens. Ovariectomy decreased their levels only slightly. Testosterone and androstenedione decreased by 40% after suppression and increased by 50% after stimulation. Ovariectomy decreased their levels by half.

The levels of oestrone and oestradiol, as well as the ratio of oestrone to androstenedione, are correlated with the weight of the woman and her fat mass. The amount of fat tissue in the post-menopausal female is apparently a major determining factor of oestrogen levels. Androstenedione is the main precursor to oestrogens. However, androstenedione levels themselves are not influenced by fat mass. It is therefore probable that the correlation between oestrogen and fat mass is a consequence of an increased androstenedione conversion in obesity. It was concluded that the post-menopausal ovary still secretes androgens (mainly testosterone) but not oestrogens.

FEMALE AND MALE CLIMACTERIC

Oestrogens originate mainly from peripheral conversion of androgens. Oestrone and oestradiol levels in the post-menopausal woman correlate with overweight and fat mass.

## HORMONE PROFILES IN POST-MENOPAUSAL WOMEN
(Introduced by H. S. Jacobs)

The hormone profiles in post-menopausal women in whom plasma samples were obtained every 20 minutes for 24 hours were reported. This technique allowed a detailed assessment to be made of unconjugated oestrogens and oestrogens and androgens. Simultaneous measurements of plasma cortisol gave an index of adrenocortical ACTH interactions. The major change when post-menopausal women were compared to pre-menopausal women was a fall of plasma oestradiol. Androstenedione concentrations showed a diurnal variation in parallel with that of cortisol. This and other parallel stress related peaks suggest an adrenal source of androstenedione.

The relationship of hormone levels to climacteric symptoms – dyspareunia and flushing attack – were investigated. When oestradiol levels were high the patient might have no symptom or flushes, but dyspareunia was seen only in patients with low oestradiol levels. There were no differences in oestrone levels. Flushing attacks could not be correlated with any specific hormone concentrations. Vaginal smear studies corroborated the finding that dyspareunia relates to low oestradiol levels.

## DISCUSSION

The general discussion underlined that during the pre-menopausal period changes occur within the ovary concerning the follicle population as well as the non-follicular tissue of the ovary which lead to marked changes in the intra-ovarian and extra-ovarian hormonal milieu. More detailed studies are needed before a complete understanding of the ageing process within the ovary and its consequences is reached.

## Bibliography

Arias, M. and Aschheim, P. (1974). Hypophysectomy and aging: primary and secondary ovarian senescence. *Experientia*, **30**, 213

Aschheim, P. (1976). Aging in the hypothalamic–hypophyseal–ovarian axis in the rat. In: *Hypothalamus, Pituitary and Aging* (A. V. Everitt and J. A. Burgess, eds.), pp. 376–418. (Springfield: Charles C. Thomas)

Chakravarti, S., Collins, W. P., Forecast, J. D., Newton, J. R., Oram, D. H. and Studd, J. W. W. (1976). Hormone profiles after the menopause. *Br. Med. J.*, **2**, 784

Crumeyrolle-Arias, M., Scheib, D. and Aschheim, P. (1976). Light and electron-microscopy of the ovarian interstitial tissue in the senile rat: Normal aspect and response to HCG of 'deficiency cells' and 'epithelial cords'. *Gerontology*, **22**, 185

Grodin, J. M., Siiteri, P. K. and McDonald, P. (1973). Source of estrogen production in postmenopausal women. *J. Clin. Endocrinol.*, **36**, 207

Harman, S. M. and Talbert, G. B. (1970). The effect of maternal age on ovulation, corpora lutea of pregnancy and implantation failure in mice. *J. Reprod. Fertil.*, **23**, 33

Hemsell, D. L., Grodin, M., Brenner, P. F., Siiteri, P. K. and McDonald, P. C. (1974). Plasma precursors of estrogen. II. Correlation of the extent of conversion of plasma androstenedione with age. *J. Clin. Endocrinol.*, **38**, 476

Judd, H. L., Lucas, W. E. and Yen, S. C. C. (1974). Effect of oophorectomy on circulating testosterone and androstenedione levels in patients with endometrial cancer. *Am. J. Obstet. Gynecol.*, **38**, 793

Judd, H. L., Judd, G. E., Lucas, W. E. and Yen, S. C. C. (1974). Endocrine function of the post-menopausal ovary: Concentration of androgen and estrogens in ovarian and peripheral vein blood. *J. Clin. Endocrinol.*, **39**, 1020

Kram, D. and Schneider, E. L. (1978). An effect of reproductive aging: Increased risk of genetically abnormal offspring. In: *The Aging Reproductive System* (Aging, Vol. 4) (E. L. Schneider, ed.) (New York: Raven Press)

Longcope, C., Pratt, J. H., Schneider, S. H. and Finberg, S. E. (1978). Aromatization of androgens by muscle and adipose tissue *in vivo*. *J. Clin. Endocrinol.*, **46**, 146

Polani, P. E. and Jagiello, G. M. (1976). Chiasmata, meiotic univalents and age in relation to aneuploid imbalance in mice. *Cytogenet. Cell Genet.*, **16**, 505

Rizkallah, T. H., Tovell, H. M. M. and Kelly, W. C. (1975). Production of estrone and fractional conversion of circulatory androstenedione to estrone in women with endometrial carcinoma. *J. Clin. Endocrinol.*, **40**, 1045

Talbert, G. B. (1977). Aging of the reproductive system. In: *Handbook of the Biology of Aging* (C. E. Finch, ed.), Vol. 3, pp. 318–356. Handbook of Aging series. (New York: Van Nostrand Reinhold)

Talbert, G. B. (1978). The effect of aging of the ovaries and female gametes on reproductive capacity. In: *The Aging Reproductive System* (E. L. Schneider, ed.) (Aging, Vol. 4), pp. 59–83 (New York: Raven Press)

Thung, P. J. (1961). Aging changes in the ovary. In: *Structural Aspects of Aging* (J. Bourne, ed.), pp. 109–142 (New York: Hafner)

Vermeulen, A. (1976). The hormonal activity of the post-menopausal ovary. *J. Clin. Endocrinol.*, **42**, 247

Vermeulen, A. and Verdonck, L. (1978). Sex hormone concentrations in post-menopausal women. *Clin. Endocrinol.* (In press)

21

---

# The climacteric syndrome

## Moderator: J. W. W. Studd

King's College Hospital Medical School, London, United Kingdom

*Participants invited to present their views at this
workshop included:*

S. Campbell (United Kingdom)
R. B. Greenblatt (USA)
A. A. Haspels (The Netherlands)
L. B. Jaszmann (The Netherlands)
D. H. Oram (South Africa)
D. W. Sturdee (United Kingdom)
M. H. Thom (United Kingdom)
W. H. Utian (USA)

The debate concerning the side-effects of oestrogen therapy for post-menopausal women is currently causing much anxiety, but of no less importance is the need for a clear understanding of the symptomatology and the endocrine changes of the climacteric syndrome. It is a truism to state that the best way to prevent complications of treatment is to withhold such treatment particularly in patients where this therapy is inappropriate. It follows that the correct selection of patients and a general agreement about symptoms which are due to oestrogen deficiency, rather than the results of the many life stresses of the middle years, is vital. Any carelessness in the criteria for treatment will lead to the misuse of oestrogen replacement therapy which will then be in danger of becoming the therapeutic crutch of stressed womankind, such as has happened with tranquillizers in the last two decades.

## SYMPTOMATOLOGY

Two milestones in the study of the climacteric were the prospective placebo trials of Utian (1972) and of Campbell (1977). The former was an extensive single-blind study assessing the true clinical effect of endogenous oestrogen withdrawal following bilateral oophorectomy and the natural menopause. In addition, the subsequent response to exogenous oestrogen therapy was determined in an attempt to differentiate this therapeutic response from a simple placebo response. It was found that hot flushes, night sweats and the symptoms of atrophic vaginitis responded to oestrogen therapy, but other symptoms such as depression, irritability, angina pectoris, insomnia and palpitations responded significantly to placebo therapy and were most likely of psychological origin. It was agreed that this excellent study would have been more valid if the assessment had been double-blind.

**Table 4.1  Symptoms significantly improved by oestrogen therapy when compared with placebo (Campbell and Whitehead, 1977)**  .

| *2-month crossover study* *(64 patients)* | *6-month crossover study* *(61 patients)* |
|---|---|
| 1.  Hot flushes | 1.  Hot flushes |
| 2.  Insomnia | 2.  Vaginal dryness |
| 3.  Vaginal dryness | 3.  Insomnia |
| 4.  Irritability | 4.  Urinary frequency |
| 5.  Poor memory | 5.  Poor memory |
| 6.  Anxiety | |
| 7.  Worry about age | |
| 8.  Headaches | |
| 9.  Worry about self | |
| 10.  Urinary frequency | |
| 11.  Optimism | |
| 12.  Good spirits | |

A double-blind protocol was used in the two studies of Campbell (1977) in which 64 patients had a 2-month crossover and 61 patients underwent a 6-month crossover study using conjugated equine oestrogens (Premarin) and a placebo tablet. A convincing placebo response was demonstrated with symptoms of vaginal dryness, coital satisfaction, urinary frequency and such elusive qualities as an improvement in memory and youthful skin appearance. This placebo effect on vaginal dryness and urinary frequency disappeared in the longer study, but the significant placebo effect on the youthful skin appearance was maintained. The clearly demonstrated benefits of oestrogen therapy in the short study were related to hot flushes, insomnia, vaginal dryness, irritability, poor memory, anxiety, 'worry about age', headaches, 'worry about self', urinary frequency and good spirits. Many of these beneficial effects were maintained and enhanced by prolonged therapy, and a significant improvement by oestrogen therapy compared with placebo in the 6-month cross-over study was found with hot flushes, vaginal dryness, insomnia and poor memory (Table 4.1). Many of these symptomatic improvements were due to the 'domino effect' whereby the cessation of vasomotor symptoms, particularly at night, enabled the patient to enjoy undisturbed sleep and a less fatigued, more efficient working and domestic life. It is the experience of the delegates that, following the correction of the oestrogen deficiency state, many patients are able to discontinue long-standing ingestion of psychoactive drugs.

A potential criticism of this convincing study is that there was no 'washout period' between the medication and the placebo courses. In order to answer this comment Campbell showed that when taking the symptoms present in the last 2 months of the two 6-month periods in the crossover study the results were still valid and, furthermore, that a beneficial effect upon libido was shown for the first time, and also a surprisingly beneficial effect upon backache.

The minor side-effects of leg cramps, breast tenderness, fluid retention, nausea, and vaginal discharge were all more commonly reported by patients during treatment with Premarin than with placebo. However, the importance of placebo in the aetiology of the side-effects was clearly demonstrated in that in every case more patients reported symptoms during the first course of treatment than during the second month.

## ENDOCRINOLOGY

The endocrinology of the climacteric was discussed by Oram who showed in his study of 60 women, 1–30 years after the normal menopause, that androstenedione, oestrone and oestradiol concentrations were reduced to about 20% of the values recorded during the early proliferative phase of the menstrual cycle. Plasma testosterone

**Table 4.2  Geometric mean concentrations (and range) of various steroids in peripheral venous plasma from post-menopausal women**

| Years after menopause | <1 | 2-3 | 5 | 10 | 20 | 30 |
|---|---|---|---|---|---|---|
| Androstenedione | 1.24 | 1.15 | 2.08 | 1.64 | 1.48 | 1.27 |
| (nmol/l) | (0.62–3.02) | (0.45–2.46) | (1.05–4.46) | (0.98–4.39) | (0.75–3.88) | (0.35–5.60) |
| Testosterone | 1.83 | 1.36 | 0.94 | 1.49 | 1.85 | 2.01 |
| (nmol/l) | (0.79–3.38) | (0.67–2.70) | (0.55–2.18) | (0.59–2.98) | (1.19–2.47) | (1.45–2.62) |
| Oestrone | 88.9 | 64.6 | 67.9 | 34.3 | 34.3 | 41.7 |
| /pmol/l | (36.9–147.6) | (36.9–92.9) | (36.9–156.8) | (9.2–101.4) | (9.2–119.3) | (27.7–73.8) |
| Oestradiol | 51.8 | 50.7 | 49.4 | 43.4 | 76.5 | 65.1 |
| (pmol/l) | (27.6–147.1) | (27.6–119.5) | (27.6–183.8) | (18.4–91.9) | (27.6–294.1) | (27.6–229.8) |

Conversion: SI to traditional units – Androstenedione: 1 nmol/l 28.6 ng/100 ml. Testosterone: 1 nmol/l 28.8 ng/100 ml. Oestrone: 1 pmol/l 0.027 ng/100 ml. Oestradiol: 1 pmol/l 0.272 ng/100 ml concentrations remained in the normal range for pre-menopausal women during these 30 years (Table 4.2). Mean concentration of follicle stimulating hormone (FSH) reached a peak of 18 times the mean proliferative stage values at 2–3 years after the menopause, and then gradually declined in the next three decades to values that were 40–50% of these maximal levels (Chakravarti *et al.*, 1976). A similar pattern of plasma hormone levels was seen for luteinizing hormone

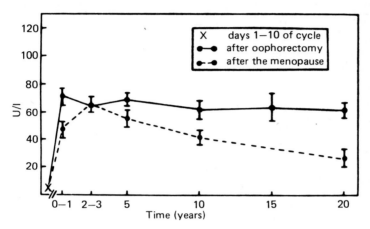

**Figure 4.1**    Plasma FSH concentration over 20 years following the natural meno-pause compared with 20 years following bilateral oophorectomy

(LH) although the peak reached was only 3.4 times that found in the first 10 days of the menstrual cycle and never reached the levels found during the pre-ovulatory surge of LH. Plasma levels of these pituitary gonadotrophins began to rise before the cessation of menstruation and if a laboratory diagnosis is, on infrequent occasions, required for the diagnosis of ovarian failure it is suggested that a single FSH assay is the most valuable.

## ENDOCRINE CHANGES AFTER BILATERAL OOPHORECTOMY

Further investigations of 100 patients from 1–20 years following bilateral oophorectomy revealed that the maximal levels of FSH and LH after castration were reached during the first year and that there was no subsequent decrease in these plasma concentrations with increasing age (Figure 4.1, Chakravarti *et al.*, 1977). Plasma oestradiol values were 80% below the mean values of days 1–10 of the menstrual cycle, and the same as would be found a comparable number of years after normal menopause. Plasma testosterone was significantly lower than after a natural menopause for the first 10 years after oophorectomy, presumably due to the loss of ovarian androgens. Vasomotor symptoms occurred shortly after surgery and there was a greater incidence in depression, dyspareunia and loss of libido than following a natural menopause. There was, however, no correlation between plasma hormone levels of FSH and testosterone and the presence or absence of vasomotor symptoms or depression (Table 4.3).

**Table 4.3 The concentration (mean and range) of various hormones in peripheral venous plasma from symptomatic oophorectomized women compared with asymptomatic oophorectomized women**

|  | *Symptomatic*<br>*(n = 66)* | *Asymptomatic*<br>*(n = 34)* |
|---|---|---|
| FSH (U/l) | 66.6<br>(35.2–140.0) | 62.4<br>(45.4–122.0) |
| LH (U/l) | 37.7<br>(10.0–78.9) | 34.6<br>(12.7–60.6) |
| Testosterone (nmol/l) | 1.09<br>(0.19–2.77) | 1.26<br>(0.46–3.07) |
| Oestradiol (pmol/l) | 61.76<br>(17.22–136.03) | 67.74<br>(34.19–104.41) |

## RECOGNITION OF ENDOGENOUS DEPRESSION IN THE CLIMACTERIC

In pre-menopausal women complaining of alleged oestrogen deficiency symptoms, a correlation was found between high plasma FSH levels and oestrogen responsive symptoms and the presence of hot flushes. FSH value of 15 IU/l was found to be a useful diagnostic cut-off point, with higher values being associated with vasomotor symptoms, and psychological and sexual symptoms responsive to endogenous oestrogen therapy. On the other hand, patients who sought oestrogen therapy for their multiplicity of psychological symptoms, and who had neither elevated FSH values nor characteristic vasomotor symptoms, did not respond to oestrogen therapy. Such patients required psychotherapy as a primary treatment. It was stated that a detailed history was essential for distinguishing patients with these symptoms of recent origin from patients with a premorbid history of affective disorder. However, it became very apparent that gynaecologists and psychiatrists pursued different lines of questioning to establish diagnosis of endogenous depression potentially treatable with anti-depressants.

## SEXUAL PROBLEMS IN THE CLIMACTERIC

Psychosexual problems were reported by Studd (1977) to occur in 45% of his clinic patients. Once again there is no correlation between plasma oestradiol, FSH and testosterone levels and the symptoms of dyspareunia or loss of libido (Table 4.4). Patients who complained of dyspareunia alone had a high (84%) incidence of vasomotor symptoms and a low (37%) incidence of anxiety, depression or irritability. These symptoms usually improved with oestrogen therapy and seemed to correspond with Utian's view of the therapeutic response to oestrogen of the classical symptoms following vaginal atrophy and vasomotor instability.

Table 4.4   Plasma testosterone and oestradiol values in groups of post-menopausal patients complaining of dyspareunia, loss of libido and dyspareunia plus loss of libido

| | Oestradiol (pmol/l) | Testosterone ($\mu$mol/l) |
|---|---|---|
| Dyspareunia | 70.6 | 1.46 |
| $n = 19$ | (34.2–161.8) | (0.51–2.72) |
| Loss of libido | 120.4 | 1.04 |
| $n = 59$ | (51.2–236.0) | (0.42–2.39) |
| Dyspareunia + | 96.2 | 1.26 |
| loss of libido | (33.2–176.4) | (0.56–2.50) |
| $n = 58$ | | |

On the other hand, the patients with the principal complaint of loss of libido had only a 38% incidence of vasomotor symptoms and a much higher than normal incidence (78%) of psychogenic symptoms. These were a more complex sub-population and the results of oestrogen replacement therapy were much less satisfactory with 76 of 117 patients complaining of a residual symptom of loss of libido. These 76 patients were given a subcutaneous hormone implant of pellets of 50 mg oestradiol and 100 mg testosterone. Only 10 patients failed to respond; 22 patients had a good response and the remaining 44 women were reported as having an excellent response meaning a return of libido as good or better than ever before.

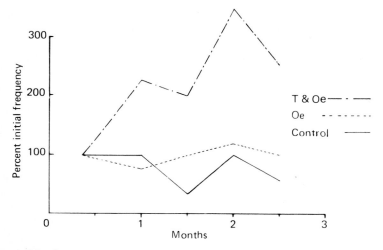

**Figure 4.2** Percentage increase in incidence of orgasm following implantation of testosterone 100 mg plus oestradiol 50 mg (T + Oe), oestradiol 30 mg (Oe) and placebo

The beneficial effects of implantation of oestradiol plus testosterone have also been demonstrated by prospective double-blind placebo trials using oestradiol, a combination of oestradiol plus testosterone, and a placebo preparation, evaluating degrees of sexual arousal, pleasure by self-rating scale and also by the frequency of masturbation, intercourse and orgasm. All of these variables had the greatest response to the combined hormone preparation (Figure 4.2).

Following oestradiol implantation, vasomotor instability was the first symptom to be relieved at about 2 to 3 weeks. An improvement of libido occurred at 6–8 weeks coincident with the time of maximal elevated plasma testosterone (Figure 4.3). The hormone implant lasted for approximately 6 months, at which time there was a fall in plasma testosterone and an elevation in plasma FSH. It was stressed that all patients with an intact uterus must have a monthly withdrawal bleeding produced by a 7–10 day course of a progestogen such as norethisterone 5 mg daily, otherwise endometrial hyperplasia and irregular uterine bleeding is inevitable. An intriguing

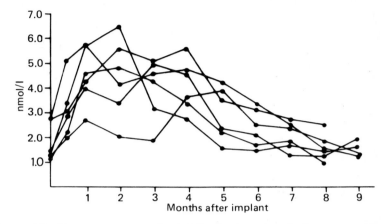

**Figure 4.3** Plasma testosterone levels following insertion of subcutaneous implant of 100 mg testosterone plus 50 mg oestradiol in six oophorectomized patients

difference in the response to oral and implant therapy is that oestradiol valerate tablets produce high levels of oestrone, but when oestradiol pellets are inserted into the body fat, thus bypassing the gastro-intestinal tract, the principal plasma oestrogen present in the plasma is oestradiol, with a ratio of oestradiol to oestrone of 2:1 (Figure 4.4).

The most characteristic of all the climacteric symptoms is the hot flush. This has been investigated by Sturdee (1978) and revealed in a pictorial fashion by thermography to demonstrate the sudden skin temperature change that occurs with flushing of the upper chest, face and neck. Eighteen hot flushes in eight menopausal women were studied. They varied in duration with a range of 1–4 minutes and intensity. In each case there was an acute rise in skin temperature which usually coincided with the subjective sensation of flushing. There was a significant increase in the heart rate at the onset of flushing but no change of cardiac rhythm. The ECG base line fluctuated considerably at the onset of flushing and this coincided

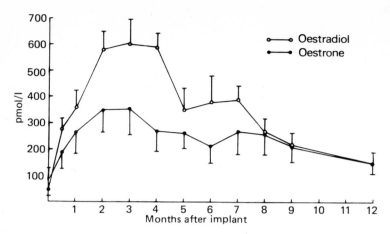

**Figure 4.4** Mean plasma oestrone and oestradiol values in 10 oophorectomized patients following subcutaneous implant of 100 mg oestradiol

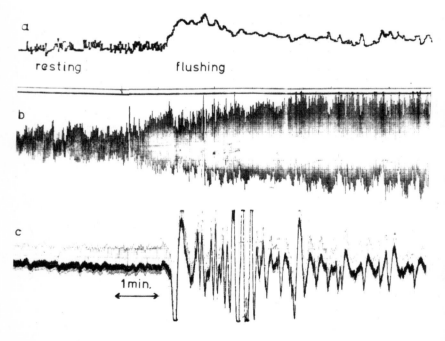

**Figure 4.5** Physiological recordings of, from top to bottom: (a) heart rate (beats per minute), (b) digital plethysmography, and (c) ECG from one menopausal woman before and during a hot flush

32

with a large increase in the digital blood volume pressure. The onset of the flush was also accompanied by an acute fall in skin resistance. The recordings of heart rate, digital plethysmography and ECG are shown in Figure 4.5. Evidence for the release of a circulating vasoactive factor was obtained by the study of blood taken before and during flushing and its contractile action on rat stomach strips following the addition of selective antagonists. This vasoactive factor apparent during a flush that was not present at other times did not appear to be 5-hydroxytryptamine, histamine, acetylcholine, kinine or catecholamines. It was agreed that this type of physiological study of the pathogenesis of vasomotor instability was of the utmost importance to enable treatment of these distressing symptoms with a non-hormonal preparation if oestrogens are for any reason contraindicated.

## References

Campbell, S. and Whitehead, M. (1977). Oestrogen therapy and the menopausal syndrome. In: *Clinics in Obstetrics and Gynaecology* (R. G. Greenblatt and J. W. W. Studd, eds.), vol. 4, pp. 31–48. (London: W. B. Saunders)

Chakravarti, S., Collins, W. P., Forecast, J. D., Utian, J. R., Oram, D. H. and Studd, J. W. W. (1976). Hormone profiles after the menopause. *Br. Med. J.*, **2**, 784

Chakravarti, S., Collins, W. P., Newton, J. R., Oram, D. H. and Studd, J. W. W. (1977). Endocrine changes after oophorectomy in premenopausal women. *Br. J. Obstet. Gynaecol.*, **84**, 769

Studd, J. W. W., Collins, W. P., Chakravarti, S., Newton, J. R., Oram, D. H. and Parsons, A. (1977). Oestradiol and testosterone implants in the treatment of psychosexual problems in the postmenopausal woman. *Br. J. Obstet. Gynaecol.*, **84**, 314

Sturdee, D. W., Wilson, K. A., Pipili, E. and Crocker, A. D. (1978). Physiological aspects of menopausal hot flush. *Br. Med. J.*, **2**, 79

Utian, W. H. (1972). The true clinical features of postmenopause and oophorectomy and their response to oestrogen therapy. *S. Afr. Med. J.*, **46**, 732

# Hypothalamic-pituitary-ovarian relationships around the menopause

## Moderator: M. Ben-David

Hebrew University, Hadassah Medical School, Jerusalem, Israel

## Secretary: P. F. A. van Look

Department of Obstetrics and Gynaecology, University Hospital, Leiden, The Netherlands

*Participants invited to present their views at this workshop included:*

*R. B. Greenblatt (USA)*
*H. S. Jacobs (United Kingdom)*
*F. Labrie (Canada)*
*P. F. A. van Look (The Netherlands)*
*H. P. G. Schneider (West Germany)*

Normal reproductive function is dependent upon the functional integrity of a delicately balanced feedback system operating between the ovaries and the hypothalamic–pituitary unit. Structural or functional disorders of either of the two components of this feedback system may upset this balance and hence lead to reproductive failure.

In the case of reproductive failure associated with ageing, there is good evidence to suggest that in laboratory species such as the rat and mouse, the decline of reproductive capacity in older females can be attributed primarily to a functional upset in hypothalamic–pituitary activity rather than to primary ovarian failure (Aschheim, 1976). The ovaries of aged, persistently oestrous or repetitive pseudopregnant rats contain a considerable number of healthy-looking primordial follicles, and when transplanted into ovariectomized, young females are quite capable of restoring regular oestrous cycles in the host. Conversely, when ovaries of young females are transplanted into elderly, ovariectomized females showing persistent oestrus or repetitive pseudopregnancies before ovariectomy, no regular oestrous cycles ensue and the recipient reverts to the irregular cycle pattern which existed before operation. From these and other studies it has been concluded that reproductive failure due to ageing in species such as the rat is due predominantly to hypothalamic–pituitary malfunctioning. The exact mechanisms responsible for this malfunctioning are at present unclear but may involve an impairment of oestrogen-induced gonadotrophin release leading to irregular cycles (Lu *et al.*, 1977) and increased sensitivity of prolactin release for oestrogen stimulation (Aschheim, 1976).

In the human (and probably also in some primate species and certain inbred strain of mice) the situation appears to be different. Unlike in the rat, hypothalamic–pituitary function does not appear to be affected by age in the majority of peri- and post-menopausal women (see below). There is, however, a marked decline in the number of primordial follicles present in the ovaries of these species so that at the end of the reproductive life-span few follicles remain. Thus primary failure of the ovaries appears to represent the key-event leading to reproductive failure in the human and a few other species. Because of the feedback relation between the ovaries and the hypothalamic–pituitary unit the decline in ovarian secretory activity which accompanies the disappearance of follicles does have important repercussions on the activity of hypothalamus and pituitary.

## HYPOTHALAMUS

The release of gonadotrophins from the anterior pituitary is stimulated by a gonadotrophin-releasing hormone (GnRH) of hypothalamic origin. The secretion of this hypothalamic neurohormone is influenced by feedback action of steroid hormones. At present no workable assay method is available to measure the concentrations of GnRH in human peripheral plasma but it is generally assumed that in post-menopausal women GnRH levels are elevated. Studies in the rhesus monkey (Carmel *et al.*, 1976) indicate that GnRH is released in a pulsatile manner from the hypothalamus into the hypophyseal vessels, and this may account for the pulsatile secretion of gonadotrophins from the pituitary (Yen *et al.*, 1972). Whether this increased secretion of GnRH in peri-menopausal women has other effects apart from the stimulatory action on pituitary gonado-trophin secretion remains uncertain.

In the rat administration of GnRH or one of its more potent agonists blocks the normal pro-oestrous rise in the number of ovarian receptors for LH and FSH. A similar reduction in gonadotrophin receptor activity, and hence probably in ovarian sensitivity to gonadotrophins, may perhaps also account for the observed prema-ture luteal regression in women treated with GnRH during the mid-luteal phase of the cycle (Labrie). Although more direct experi-mental proof is still required, it seems not unlikely from these studies that GnRH-induced gonadotrophin release may have an inhibitory effect on ovarian function. If this is so, an increased secretion of GnRH, and hence of gonadotrophins, may perhaps contribute, at least in part, to some of the abnormalities in follicular development and/or luteal function in women approaching the menopause.

It is likely that most, if not all, of the neurovegetative symptoms which are commonly associated with the menopause, originate from or are mediated through the hypothalamus, but the exact mechanisms causing these symptoms are unknown. It was generally agreed by the participants in this workshop that far more information is needed on the changes in hypothalamic neurotransmitter metab-olism around the menopause before our understanding of these symptoms is likely to improve. The observation that hot flushes in peri-menopausal women may be due to neurotransmitter substances emphasizes the need for more intensive research efforts in this area.

## PITUITARY

It is now well established that part of the feedback action of ovarian steroid hormones on gonadotrophin secretion is exerted directly at the level of the anterior pituitary. Labrie's *in vitro* studies using anterior pituitary cells in culture indicate that oestrogens stimulate the responsiveness of both FSH and LH to GnRH whereas androgens inhibit the secretion of LH but stimulate that of FSH. Progestogens, on the other hand, have a biphasic effect on LH release (stimulation followed by inhibition) but their effect on FSH secretion is exclusively stimulatory.

Apart from steroid hormones, pituitary secretion of gonadotrophins, and of FSH in particular, may also be under the control of a non-steroidal substance ('inhibin'), which has been demonstrated to be present in follicular fluid of several species (de Jong and Sharpe, 1976; Schwartz and Channing, 1977). Both *in vivo* and *in vitro* this 'inhibin-like' material has been shown to suppress preferentially the secretion of FSH.

Like most other endocrine organs the secretory activity of the pituitary gland shows very little deterioration with age. On the contrary, basal levels of FSH and LH in post-menopausal women are markedly higher than in regularly menstruating women due to the absence of negative feedback of ovarian secretory products. Apart from the rise in plasma concentrations there is an increased pituitary content of gonadotrophins and an augmented pituitary gonadotrophin response to GnRH in post-menopausal women (Schneider). In contrast to normal women in whom the repeated administration of GnRH at hourly intervals for 8 hours during the follicular phase of the cycle results eventually in a diminution of LH responses and a rise in the level of $17\beta$-oestradiol, the pituitary release of gonadotrophins following such GnRH pulses in post-menopausal women remains unchanged (Schneider).

## FEEDBACK MECHANISMS

In some peri-menopausal women it has been shown that menstrual irregularities may be due to the presence of successive waves of follicular development without intervening ovulation. The ovulatory failure of these subjects could be attributed to an impairment of LH release in response to endogenous and exogenous oestrogen stimulation (van Look *et al.*, 1977). A similar abnormality of the positive feedback system has also been described in young women with anovulatory dysfunctional bleeding (van Look *et al.*, 1978), and this defect cannot be considered, therefore, as characteristic of the menopausal age.

Most clinical studies on the effects of oestrogen or oestrogen–progestogen treatments on gonadotrophin secretion in post-menopausal women indicate that both negative and positive feedback mechanisms remain functionally intact.

## PROLACTIN

Although it is now well established that ovarian function in women of fertile age may be disturbed by hyperprolactinaemia, there is very little evidence to suggest that an increased secretion of prolactin plays a role in the decline of ovarian function at menopause. Circulating levels of prolactin in post-menopausal women are usually lower than in women of reproductive age and this may be due to the decrease in ovarian oestrogen secretion and, possibly, to an antagonism between gonadotrophin and prolactin secretion such as found in experimental animals (Ben David et al., 1971; Yarkoni et al., 1977). However, Schneider was unable to find any evidence for such antagonism in his studies on the effects of drug-induced hyperprolactinaemia on pulsatile gonadotrophin secretion in post-menopausal women.

## CHANGES IN CIRCULATING LEVELS OF GONADOTROPHINS DURING MENOPAUSAL TRANSITION

The typical hormonal changes which occur during menopausal transition in the human female can be summarized as follows (Sherman et al., 1976; van Look et al., 1977).

In women between the ages of 45 and 50 years a characteristic finding which appears to represent the hallmark of declining ovarian function is the presence of an elevated level of FSH with normal LH. This monotropic increase of FSH may be associated with a shortening of the follicular phase. The mechanism responsible for the elevated concentration of FSH is not yet fully understood but may involve a decrease in the ovarian secretion of 'inhibin-like' material of follicular origin.

When the ovarian follicle population becomes markedly reduced the interval between successive waves of follicle growth increases and menstrual bleeding becomes progressively more irregular. During periods of relative ovarian inactivity and low oestrogen secretion plasma levels of both FSH and LH are elevated to values which are intermediate between the normal and post-menopausal range but they may subsequently return to normal when follicle(s) start(s) growing. Anovulatory cycles are common in these women but they do not appear to result from a failure of positive feedback but rather from inadequate follicular oestrogen secretion.

Finally, when all gonadotrophin-sensitive follicles have disappeared from the ovaries the plasma concentration of 17$\beta$-oestradiol declines and the levels of gonadotrophins rise towards the post-menopausal range.

The various patterns of menstrual dysfunction and associated hormonal changes that have been described in peri-menopausal women have also been observed in young women receiving external irradiation or cytotoxic therapy for lymphoreticular diseases (Jacobs). This indicates that when the ovary is damaged all of the endocrine consequences of spontaneous ovarian failure can be reproduced, and hence confirms the view that in women the initial change at menopause is in the ovary and the elevations in gonadotrophin secretion are secondary to ovarian involution.

## References

Aschheim, P. (1976). Ageing in the hypothalamic–hypophyseal–ovarian axis in the rat. In: *Hypothalamus, Pituitary and Ageing* (A. V. Everett and J. A. Burgess, eds.), pp. 376–418 (Springfield: Charles C. Thomas)

Ben-David, M., Danon, A. and Sulman, F. G. (1971). Evidence of antagonism between prolactin and gonadotrophin secretion: Effect of methallibure on perphenazine-induced prolactin secretion in ovariectomized rats. *J. Endocrinol.*, **51**, 719

Carmel, P. W., Araki, S. and Ferin, M. (1976). Pituitary stalk portal blood collection in rhesus monkeys: Evidence for pulsatile release of gonadotrophin-releasing hormone (GnRH). *Endocrinology*, **99**, 243

de Jong, F. H. and Sharpe, R. M. (1976). Evidence for inhibin-like activity in bovine follicular fluid. *Nature*, **263**, 71

van Look, P. F. A., Hunter, W. M., Fraser, I. S. and Baird, D. T. (1978). Impaired estrogen-induced luteinizing hormone release in young women with anovulatory dysfunctional uterine bleeding. *J. Clin. Endocrinol.*, **46**, 816

van Look, P. F. A., Lothian, H., Hunter, W. M., Michie, E. A. and Baird, D. T. (1977). Hypothalamic–pituitary–ovarian function in perimenopausal women. *Clin. Endocrinol.*, **7**, 13

Lu, K. H., Huang, H. H., Chen, H. T., Kurcz, M., Mioduszewski, R. and Meites, J. (1977). Positive feedback by estrogen and progesterone on LH release in old and young rats. *Proc. Soc. Exp. Biol. (N.Y.)*, **154**, 82

Schwartz, N. B. and Channing, C. P. (1977). Evidence for ovarian 'inhibin':

Suppression of the secondary rise in serum follicle stimulating hormone levels in proestrous rats by injection of porcine follicular fluid. *Proc. Nat. Acad. Sci. (Wash.)*, **74**, 5721

Sherman, B. M., West, J. H. and Korenman, S. G. (1976). The menopausal transition: Analysis of LH, FSH, estradiol and progesterone concentrations during menstrual cycles of older women. *J. Clin. Endocrinol.*, **42**, 629

Yarkoni, S., Polistuk, W. Z., Spitz, I. M. and Ben-David, M. (1977). Inhibitory effect of hyperprolactinemia on induction of ovulation by gonadotropins. *Fertil. Steril.*, **28**, 772

Yen, S. S. C., Tsai, C. C., Naftolin, F., Vandenberg, G. and Ajabor, L. (1972). Pulsatile patterns of gonadotrophin release in subjects with and without ovarian function. *J. Clin. Endocrinol.*, **34**, 671

41

# Effects, side-effects, and dosage schemes of various sex hormones in the peri- and post-menopause

## Moderator: H. Kopera

Department of Experimental and Clinical Pharmacology,
University of Graz, Austria

*Participants invited to present their views at this
workshop included:*

*M. Dhont (Belgium)*
*F. Dienstl (Austria)*
*R. D. Gambrell (USA)*
*G. S. Gordan (USA)*
*J. Heidenreich (West Germany)*
*U. Lachnit-Fixon (West Germany)*
*C. Lauritzen (West Germany)*
*P. E. Lebech (Denmark)*
*R. L. Sitruk-Ware (France)*
*W. H. Utian (USA)*

Discussions at this workshop were not limited to peri-menopausal complaints, but covered also post-menopausal disturbances. Considering the diversity of opinions and experience of the many students of sex hormone treatment in the climacteric, and assuming it would be unrealistic to expect that a reasonable overall picture of the subject could be obtained in a free discussion, several experts in the field were invited to introduce the most relevant topics. These

43

presentations were subsequently commented upon and/or supplemented by the audience.

The first part of the workshop was devoted to the pharmacological possibilities available for the treatment of peri- and post-menopausal changes. In the second part the subject was approached more from the clinical point of view. A considerable though not necessarily disturbing overlapping was, of course, inherent in such a procedure.

This report summarizes the introductory speeches of the principal speakers, which stand as pars-pro-toto for the respective topics. Important contributions made during the discussions are incorporated.

---

## Therapeutic possibilities for the treatment of menopausal and post-menopausal symptoms with sex hormones

---

## PROGESTOGENS ONLY (Introduced by R. L. Sitruk-Ware)

The menopause is preceded by 6–8 years of irregular menstrual cycles and by a decline of fertility following a reduction in the number of oocytes (pre-menopause). The hormonal pattern observed during this transitional period consists of a rise in FSH concentration whilst the midcycle LH peak is either absent or delayed. The ovarian function is characterized by a normal oestradiol production in the follicular phase and normal or elevated oestradiol levels in the luteal phase when ovulation occurs. Progesterone production is uniformly low or absent as in the frequently occurring anovulatory cycles (Figure 6.1).

This disequilibrium between the oestradiol and the progesterone production is thought to be of pathophysiological importance for the appearance of several pre-menstrual complaints, such as pre-menstrual tension, mastodynia and irregular bleedings. Moreover, this hormonal imbalance seems to contribute to the pathogenesis of benign breast diseases and endometrial hyperplasia.

Recent findings indicate that progesterone and progestogens counteract the action of oestradiol in three different ways: (a) by

44

stimulating the activity of oestradiol-17$\beta$ dehydrogenase, which accelerates the conversion of oestradiol to oestrone, (b) by decreasing the number of oestradiol receptors, and (c) by inhibiting epithelial cell growth and taking cells out of the cell cycle and putting them in a resting period.

It seems justified to assume that pre-menopausal complaints may be relieved by correcting the progesterone insufficiency during the

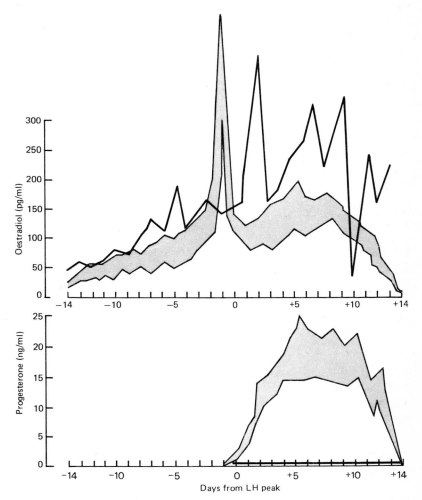

**Figure 6.1** Anovulatory cycle: Daily concentrations of serum $E_2$ and P in one subject aged 48 with infrequent menses compared to the mean $\pm$ 2 SEM in normal cycles (shaded area)

presumed luteal phase, with the aim of restoring the diminished progestational activity, and of producing an antioestrogenic effect at the target level. When selecting suitable compounds the progestational activity, the antioestrogenic properties, the gonado-trophin-inhibiting and thus contraceptive effect, and the incidence of side-effects produced are of importance; furthermore, the compound should have no androgenic action, no glucocorticoid effect but possibly an antimineralocorticoid activity.

To prove this assumption a trial was performed in 241 women. They were treated for various peri-menopausal complaints with lynoestrenol on a sequential basis. The best results were obtained in connection with bleeding irregularities, mastodynia, and anxiety; less impressive results were observed in connection with fibrocystic disease and cyclic oedemas (Table 6.1). In the discussion it was suggested that all these conditions might also be treated with either a combination of an oestrogen and an androgen or of an oestrogen and a progestogen.

Table 6.1   Results of the treatment of peri-menopausal complaints in 241 patients with a sequential regimen of lynoestrenol

| Symptoms | Number of patients | Successes (%) | Failures (%) |
|---|---|---|---|
| Mastodynia | 200 | 85.5 | 14.5 |
| Pre-menstrual tension with anxiety | 180 | 89 | 11 |
| Cyclic oedemas | 20 | 10 | 90 |
| Irregular vaginal bleeding | 198 | 97 | 3 |
| Benign breast diseases fibrocystic disease | 62 | 40 | 60 |

# OESTROGENS PLUS ANDROGENS AND OESTROGENS PLUS PROGESTATIVES (Introduced by U. Lachnit-Fixon)

## Oestrogen-androgen preparations

In the 1950s combined oestrogen–androgen preparations were developed with the objective of intensifying the desired effect of oestrogens on climacteric complaints and at the same time of minimizing their action on the endometrium. Various short- and long-chain esters of testosterone and oestradiol were combined in preparations mainly for intra-muscular administration. They were found to be very effective, particularly for psychic symptoms such as depressive mood, but untoward side-effects such as virilization and the fact that patients became almost addicted to the androgen medication resulted in these preparations being used less and less, and nowadays they are administered when treatment with oestrogens alone or in combination with progestogens fails. There is one combination, however, viz.: oestradiol valerate with prasterone oenanthate, a sexually unspecific steroid, which seems to be effective without any apparent risk of virilization.

The meeting discussed whether anabolic steroids, because of their lower androgenic potency, could possibly replace androgens, but no conclusions were reached because of a lack of experience.

## Oestrogen–progestogen preparations

Replacement therapy with strong endometriotrophic oestrogens alone produces prolonged unopposed oestrogen action resulting in endometrial hyperplasia, which can be a 'terrain factor' for neoplastic growth. Therefore, oral two-phase oestrogen–progestogen preparations enjoy increasing attention for the therapy of peri- and post-menopausal disturbances. The overstimulation of the target organ is prevented by the antiproliferative effect of the progestogen, and the endometrium is normally transformed and regularly shed if the preparations are taken cyclically. The addition of a progestogen to oestrogen therapy is particularly recommended in women with risk factors for endometrial carcinoma.

Two-phase oestrogen–progestogen preparations are very effective in controlling climacteric complaints, produce but few side-effects and consequently have become part of the routine therapy for climacteric symptoms.

## CONJUGATED OESTROGENS WITH AND WITHOUT PROGESTOGENS (Introduced by R. D. Gambrell)

The results obtained with conjugated oestrogens alone and in combination with progestogens were demonstrated by presenting the results of a very extensive current study involving, to date, 5880 patient years of observation in women with an intact uterus.

Of the women involved 64.5% were treated with an oestrogen–progestogen combination, the progestogen being added in order to prevent adenocarcinoma of the endometrium. The progestogens have been seen to be effective in that the incidence of endometrial cancer in the oestrogen–progestogen users was 0.3 : 1000 women per year and 3.8 : 1000 women per year in those taking oestrogens only (Table 6.2).

**Table 6.2   Incidence of endometrial cancer at Wilford Hall USAF Medical Center: 1975–1977**

|  | Patient-years of observation | Cancers | Incidence |
|---|---|---|---|
| Oestrogen users | 2088 | 8 | 3.8 : 1000 |
| Oestrogen–progestogen users | 3792 | 1 | 0.3 : 1000 |
| Other hormones* | 775 | 1 | 1.3 : 1000 |
| Untreated women | 1515 | 3 | 2.0 : 1000 |
| TOTAL | 8170 | 13 | 1.6 : 1000 |

* Oestrogen vaginal cream, progestogens, androgens (1976–1977)

The major side-effect of the added progestogen is the occurrence of withdrawal bleedings, which occur in 97% of the oestrogen–progestogen post-menopausal women, but in only 33.7% of those treated with conjugated oestrogens alone. However, only 0.9% of the oestrogen–progestogen users had irregular bleedings, against 21% of those taking only conjugated oestrogens.

The incidence of breast cancer is lower in patients taking conjugated oestrogens only when compared to untreated women (Table 6.3). The addition of a progestogen apparently does not further decrease the incidence of breast cancer in oestrogen-treated women. During 14 548 total patient years of observation, which includes patients that have had a hysterectomy and therefore not at risk for endometrial cancer, 48 breast cancers were diagnosed for an overall incidence of 3.3 : 1000 women per year.

Other side-effects of conjugated oestrogens–progestogens therapy include oedema, bloating, increased irritability pre-menstrually, lower abdominal cramps, dysmenorrhoea, and breast tenderness. Oedema, bloating and irritability are more frequent in women receiving conjugated oestrogens therapy alone. These symptoms are best managed by decreasing the oestrogen dosage and adding diuretics. Lower abdominal cramps during progestogen therapy and dysmenorrhoea are best managed with analgesics or by changing treatment to another progestogen. The analgesic prescribed should include aspirin because of its prostaglandin-inhibiting properties since prostaglandins are related to the uterine cramps that produce the dysmenorrhoea.

Dydrogesterone seems to be the most effective progestogen for preventing dysmenorrhoea. Breast tenderness and aggravation of fibrocystic disease are best managed by decreasing the oestrogen dosage and adding medroxyprogesterone acetate, even for hysterectomized women.

Dosage schemes for conjugated oestrogens and progestogens are as follows. For women with a natural menopause, conjugated oestrogens 0.625 mg are prescribed from the first through the 25th of each month. With a surgical menopause, higher doses of conjugated oestrogens are usually needed for the first year or two following removal of the ovaries. Conjugated oestrogens 1.25 mg, also from the first through the 25th of the month, are started immediately following hysterectomy and bilateral oophorectomy. Progestogens from the 16th through the 25th of the month are given to all women with an intact uterus and to hysterectomized patients developing

**Table 6.3  Incidence of breast cancer at Wilford Hall USAF Medical Center: 1975–1977**

|  | Patient-years of observation | Cancers | Incidence |
|---|---|---|---|
| Oestrogen users | 7263 | 13 | 1.8 : 1000 |
| Oestrogen–progestogen users | 3855 | 6 | 1.6 : 1000 |
| Other hormones* | 994 | 1 | 1.0 : 1000 |
| Untreated women | 2436 | 28 | 11.5 : 1000 |
| TOTAL | 14 548 | 48 | 3.3 : 1000 |

* Oestrogen vaginal cream, progestogens, androgens (1976–1977)

breast tenderness during oestrogen therapy. Dosages of progestogens employed are norethindrone acetate 5 mg, medroxyprogesterone acetate 10 mg, or dydrogesterone 10 mg, for the last 10 days of oestrogen therapy. Conjugated oestrogens vaginal cream 1 g thrice weekly is given to older post-menopausal women with atrophic or senile vaginitis.

It was emphasized that breast cancer and a history of thrombo-embolism are contraindications for oestrogen therapy.

**Table 6.4  Oestrogen doses required for disappearance of sweating and flushes**

| Oestrogen dose | Mode of administration | No. of subjects | Period of treatment (Years) | | Side-effects | | | | |
|---|---|---|---|---|---|---|---|---|---|
| | | | Mean | Range | Oedema | Weight gain | Nausea, headache | Other | Total |
| Oestradiol 1 mg } | Cont. | 0 | 2.6 | (1–5) | 0 | 0 | 0 | 0 | 0 |
| Oestriol 0.5 mg } | Cycl. | 6 | | | | | | | |
| Oestradiol 2 mg } | Cont. | 20 | — | — | 3 | 2 | 0 | 4 | 6 |
| Oestriol 1 mg } | Cycl. | 72 | | | | | | | |
| Oestradiol 4 mg } | Cont. | 51 | — | — | 6 | 3 | 4 | 8 | 14 |
| Oestriol 2 mg } | Cycl. | 39 | | | | | | | |
| Oestradiol 6 mg } | Cont. | 8 | — | — | 0 | 0 | 0 | 2 | 2 |
| Oestriol 3 mg } | Cycl. | 0 | | | | | | | |
| 'Trisequence'* | | 67 | 1.9 | (1–3) | 2 | 0 | 0 | 2 | 4 |

* 12 tablets with oestradiol 2 mg plus oestriol 1 mg
10 tablets with the same oestrogens plus norethisterone acetate 1 mg
6 tablets with oestradiol 1 mg plus oestriol 0.5 mg

## NON-STEROIDAL OESTROGENS AND OESTRADIOL
(Introduced by P. E. Lebech)

Non-steroidal and synthetic steroidal oestrogens cause a variety of unwanted side-effects including untoward effects on plasma lipids, insulin, growth hormone, prolactin and thyroxine. Furthermore they are not metabolized, and are strongly bound to the receptors. Their use for the treatment of climacteric complaints is therefore discouraged.

Preference is given to natural oestrogens. Combinations of various doses of micronized oestradiol-17$\beta$ and oestriol have been found to be very effective in alleviating climacteric symptoms. They have favourable metabolic effects and cause only few undesired side-effects (Table 6.4). The combination of natural oestrogens (oestradiol plus oestriol) and a progestogen given in a sequential regimen seems to be even better. However, the opinion that this would be the most natural substitution therapy was not uniformly accepted. Discussants questioned the rationale of substitution therapy for climacteric complaints with the aim of restoring pre-climacteric endocrine conditions.

## OESTRIOL (Introduced by C. Lauritzen)

Oestriol is the main metabolite of both oestradiol and oestrone. It is a rather weak oestrogen with a spectrum of effects somewhat different from that of other oestrogens.

The main advantage of oestriol over oestrone, 17$\beta$-oestradiol, and their derivatives, is that it has only a weak endometriotrophic effect, thus its administration does not lead to endometrial hyperproliferation. It may be that, because of this, the co-carcinogenicity of oestriol is less than that of the other oestrogens. It may also be that, for the same reason, oestriol can be administered continuously.

Although the effect of oestriol on the endometrium is less than that of other oestrogens, its effect on the cervix, vagina, vulva, urethra, urinary bladder and epidermis is the same, whether administered orally, parenterally or locally. Oestriol has no apparent undesired metabolic effects on liver enzymes, coagulation factors, glucose metabolism, body weight, blood pressure, or plasma hormone binding globulins. It has a weak antigonadotrophic effect and has been found in animal experiments to have a strong antiandrogenic

51

effect. Animal experiments have also shown that at the uterine level oestriol exerts a competitive inhibition with oestrone and $17\beta$-oestradiol.

On the basis of these advantages the indications for therapy with oestriol can be rather well defined, and its use can be advocated for:

(a) patients with low- or medium-grade climacteric complaints and absence of depressive symptoms;
(b) patients in whom uterine bleedings are not desired (who had several curettages or who have a special predisposition to unwanted uterine bleedings);
(c) patients in whom the metabolic effects of oestrogens have to be avoided;
(d) patients with relative contraindications to oestrogens, such as hypertension, hypertriglyceridaemia, diabetes mellitus, an inclination to weight increase, and low-importance risk factors for thrombosis, fibromyomata, mastopathia, endometrial or mammary carcinoma after initial treatment with good prognosis.

**Table 6.5   Usual daily doses of oral oestriol or oestriol succinate necessary to improve low- and medium-grade climacteric symptoms (continuous treatment)**

| Symptoms | Dose during the first week (mg/day) | Maintenance dose (mg/day) |
|---|---|---|
| Hot flushes, sweating | 6–8 | 2–4 |
| Atrophy of the vulva Atrophic vaginitis Atrophic urethro-cystitis Urinary stress incontinence | 2–3 | 2 |
| Calcium loss | 8–12 | 6–8 |

In Table 6.5 the daily doses of oestriol or oestriol succinate usually given orally and continuously for the treatment of climacteric symptoms are listed. Should higher doses be required, a change-over to another oestrogen is recommended.

The results of a controlled trial with two doses of oestriol and a placebo are summarized in Tables 6.6 and 6.7.

Oestriol also has disadvantages when compared to oestrone and

17$\beta$-oestradiol and their derivatives. It has weaker therapeutic effects on hot flushes and sweating and on other vegetative symptoms. It has only a weak psychotrophic effect. Its effect on the calcium balance – and therefore its antiosteoporotic effect – is not strong. Oestriol is a poor inhibitor of gonadotrophin secretion and does not inhibit ovulation. It does not stabilize the menstrual cycle.

**Table 6.6   Double-blind study with oestriol 2 mg ($n = 24$) and 4 mg ($n = 24$) against placebo ($n = 24$) in patients with medium- and low-grade climacteric complaints (continuous medication, random allocation to treatment)**

| Symptoms | % of patients with symptoms before treatment | % of symptoms abolished or improved after 8 weeks' treatment | | |
|---|---|---|---|---|
| | | 2 mg* once a day | 4 mg† once a day | placebo‡ once a day |
| Hot flushes | 83 | 74 | 85 | 18 |
| Sweating | 61 | 70 | 81 | 10 |
| Nervousness and irritability | 50 | 54 | 59 | 12 |
| Depressive mood | 32 | 62 | 60 | 5 |
| Sleeplessness | 29 | 38 | 43 | 8 |
| Atrophic colpitis | 30 | 100 | 100 | 0 |
| Atrophic urethro-cystitis | 7 | 90 | 100 | 0 |

*During the first week 6 mg/day
†During the first week 12 mg/day
‡During the first week 1 tablet t.i.d.

Significances: 2 mg oestriol versus placebo: all complaints $p < 0.001$
4 mg oestriol versus placebo: all complaints $p < 0.001$

**Table 6.7   Side-effects of oestriol and placebo treatment (trial as described in Table 6.5)**

| Side-effect | Before therapy (%) | After 1 week of therapy (%) | After 8 weeks of therapy (%) | After 8 weeks on placebo* (%) |
|---|---|---|---|---|
| Nausea | 1 | 6 | 0 | 2 |
| Gastro-intestinal symptoms | 5 | 8 | 1 | 2 |
| Oedema | 3 | 9 | 1 | 1 |
| Breast symptoms | 5 | 17 | 2 | 3 |
| Headache | 11 | 12 | 3 | 3 |
| Weight increase | 5 | 15 | 8 | 4 |
| Cervical hypersecretion | 0 | 11 | 4 | 0 |
| Leg cramps | 0 | 2 | 0 | 0 |

*The differences of the side-effects after 8 weeks' oestrogen treatment versus placebo are not significant

Because of the profile of its properties, oestriol should preferably be used for an individual therapy in patients with low- and medium-grade climacteric complaints, in particular when uterine bleedings and the metabolic effects of oestrogen are to be avoided.

---

## Menopausal and post-menopausal syndromes and their treatment with sex hormones

---

### THE NEUROVEGETATIVE MENOPAUSAL SYNDROME
(Introduced by W. H. Utian)

The following definitions were formulated at the 1st International Congress on the Menopause (1976):

(a) The climacteric is the phase in the ageing process marking the transition from the reproductive stage of life to the non-reproductive stage.

(b) Menopause indicates the final menstrual period and usually occurs between the ages of 45 and 55 with an average of 51 years.

(c) The climacteric is sometimes but not always associated with symptomatology. When this occurs the symptomatology may be termed the climacteric syndrome.

Climacteric symptoms and complaints are derived from three main factors:

(1) Decreased ovarian activity, with subsequent hormonal deficiency, resulting in early symptoms such as hot flushes, perspiration, 'night sweats', and atrophic vaginitis, and late symptoms related to the metabolic changes in the end organs.

(2) Socio-cultural factors, determined by the woman's environment.

(3) Psychological factors, dependent on the structure of the woman's character.

The variety in symptomatology is the result of interaction between these three compounds.

54

Early symptoms of oestrogen deficiency are amenorrhoea, hot flushes and perspiration ('night sweats') a later one is vaginal atrophy causing dyspareunia, etc. Contrary to popular opinion these are the only true direct hormonal-related changes in the peri-menopause. Therefore, they are the only true indications for oestrogen therapy. Many reports testify to the use of various oestrogens for the relief of peri-menopausal symptoms. Despite this there is a remarkable lack of controlled clinical trials and the choice of therapy has still to be based on relatively uncontrolled collective experience. According to present knowledge, specific oestrogen related symptoms react adequately to oestrogens and should be treated with oestrogen replacement therapy.

No evidence exists as to the relation between increased gonado-trophic output and the development of hot flushes. Oestrogen deficiency appears to be the direct factor, but the mechanism remains unexplained. Oestrogen therapy in normal clinical doses does not reduce raised FSH or LH values to pre-menopausal levels yet is sufficient to alleviate the symptoms of hot flushes.

All other symptoms usually ascribed to the climacteric (also called the 'neurovegetative menopausal syndrome') such as head-ache, fatigue, depressive mood, irritability, loss of libido, palpi-tations, and angina pectoris, are most likely part of the psycho-socio-cultural phenomena and general ageing changes occurring at this time. At any rate, there is no proof that they justify hormone replacement therapy.

Prior to treating any non-specific symptom ascribed to 'meno-pause', every effort should be undertaken to exclude organic disease that may generate such a symptom. Where oestrogen administration is indicated the type and dosage is of importance. It should be borne in mind that contraindications to oestrogen do exist; they include a history of venous thrombosis, family history of or treated breast carcinoma, liver dysfunction or chronic gallbladder disease, familial hypercholesterolaemia and porphyria.

## THE ORGANIC POST-MENOPAUSAL SYNDROME
(Introduced by J. Heidenreich)

After spontaneous or induced menopause a marked reduction of the epidermal thickness and low frequency of mitosis in the epidermis have been found. These changes in the female skin react promptly to oestrogen therapy, which restores thickness and frequency of mitosis in the epidermis and exerts a favourable influence upon the elasticity and blood circulation in the skin.

There is no acute change in the vaginal epithelium after menopause but gradually the epithelium becomes increasingly atrophic until it consists of a small basal layer only. These atrophic changes manifest themselves clinically by an increased liability to infection,

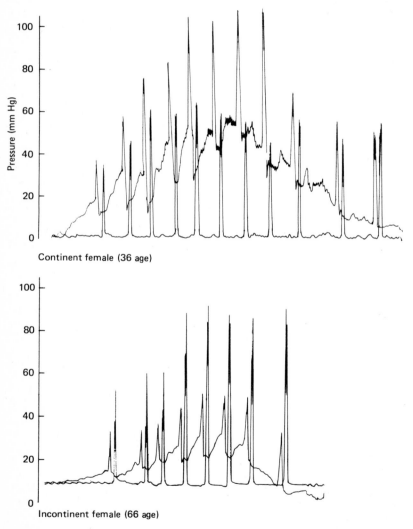

**Figure 6.2** Urethral pressure profile under stress (coughing)

56

by bleeding after minor trauma, and by dyspareunia. Oestrogen therapy readily reverses these histological abnormalities and alleviates clinical symptoms.

Oestrogen deficiency also causes atrophic changes in the urethra

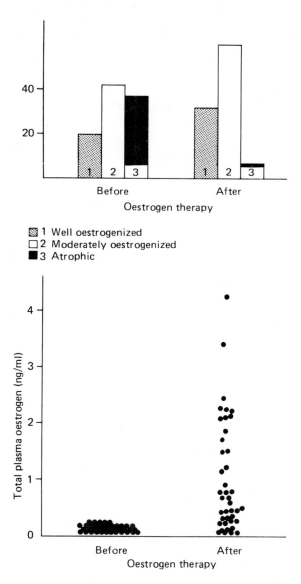

**Figure 6.3**  Cytological oestrogen assessment in the post-menopause

and urinary bladder, which are found in a very high percentage of post-menopausal women. Besides atrophic cystitis and urethritis, a loss of the tonus of the urinary bladder and urinary incontinence are found with increasing frequency. Incontinence is generally thought to be the result of a decreased urethral pressure profile with progressing age. This decrease is due, at least in part, to the diminished thickness of the peri-urethral tissue, its turgor and its vascularity. The pressure profile can be investigated with urethro-cystotonometry. Urinary continence means that the pressure within the bladder at rest as well as during stress does not exceed the maximal urethral pressure. In the case of urinary incontinence, however, the pressure in the bladder exceeds the opposing urethral resistance causing urine excretion (Figure 6.2).

The effectiveness of an oestrogen therapy on this condition was investigated with the help of urethral pressure studies in 40 patients with mostly moderate degree stress incontinence. Measurements were made before and 1 month after therapy with 2 or 4 mg oestriol daily.

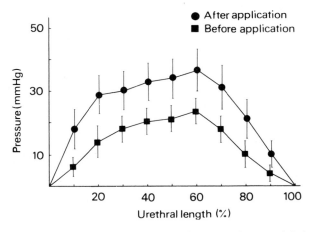

**Figure 6.4**  Urethral pressure profile before and after oestriol therapy

Due to their common origin in the urogenital sinus both vagina and urethra are very similar with regard to the squamous epithelium. Thus cytological investigation of the urinary tract is also a useful method to assess an oestrogen effect in post-menopausal women. Using the method of Papanicolaou, the cytology of urethral smears before and during or after therapy can be compared (Figure 6.3).

As a result of oestriol therapy, a statistically significant rise of the urethral pressure profile and a concomitant improvement of the urinary incontinence could be demonstrated with urethro-cysto-tonometry (Figures 6.4 and 6.5).

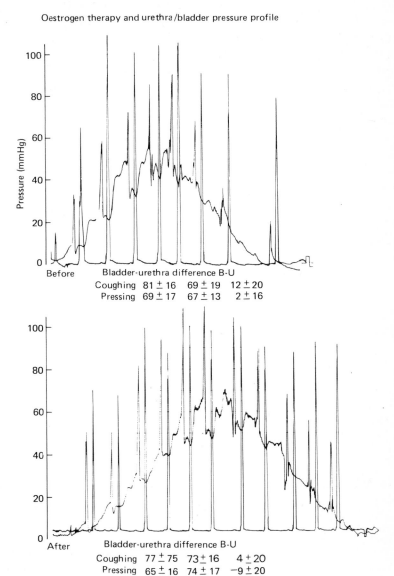

Oestrogen therapy and urethra/bladder pressure profile

**Figure 6.5** Oestrogen therapy and urethra/bladder pressure profile

59

Usually patients with an improved incontinence also show more frequently oestrogen-induced changes of the urethral smear (Figure 6.6).

The available experience favours the following conclusion: Hormonal substitution therapy with oestrogens should be tried before surgical intervention in cases of moderate degree urinary incontinence when there are other symptoms of oestrogen deficiency and when other causes for the incontinence have been excluded. Furthermore, oestrogens should be administered as a supportive measure following all incontinence operations in post-menopausal women.

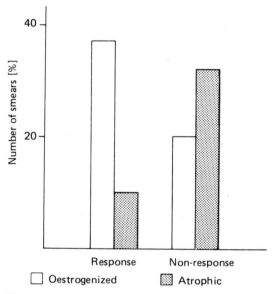

**Figure 6.6** Urethral smears in incontinence patients who improved under oestriol therapy and in those who did not

## THE METABOLIC POST-MENOPAUSAL SYNDROME
(Introduced by M. Dhont on behalf also of D. Vandekerckhove, R. Demol, M. Lemaire, Ph. Buytaert and H. Wauters)

Various metabolic changes occur in the post-menopause: plasma levels of lipoproteins and cholesterol increase, there is a tendency to obesity, and the connective tissue weakens, resulting in prolapse of the uterus and of the vagina.

Oestrogen deficiency is regarded as one of the causative factors in these multiconditional changes. Consequently, oestrogen supplementation is frequently employed to combat some of the post-menopausal metabolic disturbances. The metabolic effects of oestrogens depend on the dose administered. Administration of even low doses of synthetic oestrogens may cause hypertriglyceridaemia, and conjugated oestrogens in therapeutic doses may have a similar effect in subjects with a family history of elevated serum triglycerides. Regular respective controls are therefore recommended in such women.

The influence of oestrogens on the cholesterol level is also dose-dependent. Higher doses decrease serum cholesterol. Oestriol in a dose of 4–6 mg per day given during 3 months changes neither serum triglycerides nor the cholesterol level. However, the cholesterol phospholipid ratio decreases, i.e. it changes favourably. Free testosterone, cortisol and thyroxin do not seem to increase under oestrogen therapy.

Some groups of oestrogen treated patients have a lower relative body weight (i.e. in relation to their optimum weight) than untreated controls. However, no effect on body weight is seen in normal weight ovariectomized patients, whereas in obese women the body weight tends to decrease in the course of an adequate oestrogen therapy.

Oestrogens are said to be used frequently in older patients not only post-operatively to improve tissue repair but also pre-operatively to facilitate surgical intervention. It has been found that 20 mg oestriol per day for 2–4 weeks pre-operatively has a beneficial effect on the lower genital tract in that it changes the condition of the tissue favourably: the supporting connective tissue stands stretching better, vascularization is improved, and the sub-epithelial stroma is increased; furthermore, the epithelial layers of the lower genital tract thicken and become less fragile.

In vaginal surgery the post-operative administration of oestrogens has a beneficial effect on the healing process and on scar formation.

## THE PSYCHIC MENOPAUSAL AND POST-MENOPAUSAL SYNDROME (Introduced by H. Kopera)

Many climacteric women suffer not only from functional and organic disorders but also from widely differing psychic complaints such as listlessness, loss of concentration, diminished mental performance, irritability, aggressiveness, fatigue, emotional instability, tension, depressed mood, introversion, frustration, feelings of uselessness, and a fear of being alone. Of course, it must be remembered that at this time of her life a woman has to cope with a variety of problems. These include the cessation of the regular menses, loss of fertility, and the fear of becoming physically unattractive; in addition, in this period children marry or leave the parental home for other reasons; also at the time many women become increasingly afraid of serious illness, a fear which is made worse as one begins to lose friends and relatives through death. These and many other problems can evoke abnormal psychic reactions, the consequences of which may vary from marital troubles to antisocial behaviour.

It is evident that in the climacteric a woman has to cope with a great many fundamental changes in her social and private life. Consequently, psychic disturbances occurring in these years are to a great extent only indirectly and sometimes not at all connected with progressive oestrogen deficiency. Nevertheless, the role played by the hormonal imbalance becomes increasingly evident.

In the last few years a number of investigations have been performed to study the influence of drugs, and in particular of oestrogens, upon psychic changes. In most trials use has been made of reproducible psychometric methods, and a number of which

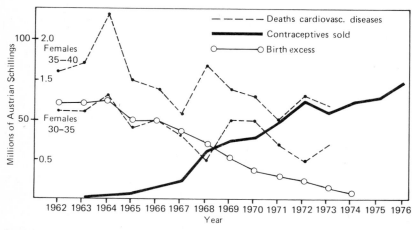

**Figure 6.7** Deaths due to cardiovascular disease in Austria in the years 1962–1973. The graph shows the increasing use of oral contraceptives and the decreasing birth excess

have fully met the requirements of accepted clinical pharmacological investigations. Reports of such investigations have clearly indicated the beneficial prophylactic, as well as therapeutic, effect of oestrogen treatment on some psychic disorders. Improvements have been seen in concentration, irritability, and on some parameters of alertness, and some reports have suggested that oestrogen therapy has prevented expected deterioration of mental performance and even reversed certain adverse changes which had already occurred.

Several discussants emphasized the importance of treating psychic disturbances in post-menopausal women and reported on the beneficial effects of oestrogens in this connection. In particular, a mood elevating, psychotonic effect, frequently resulting in a sense of extreme well-being and vigour, most probably due to restorement of somatic efficiency and psychic equilibrium, was mentioned as an effect of oestrogen substitution.

## POST-MENOPAUSAL CARDIOVASCULAR CHANGES
(Introduced by F. Dienstl)

The changes in the extent of cardiovascular risk following menopause is a controversial issue. There are several population studies which provide evidence that menopause alters this risk. Many investigators have speculated about unknown protective effects or factors in pre-menopausal women.

Menopause occurring at the normal age brings an immediate higher risk for coronary heart disease (CHD). This is detected mostly from epidemiological studies. Furthermore, there is rather strong evidence that premature menopause can lead to premature CHD. Whenever oestrogens are used for the compensation of hormonal deficiency, the potential risks of oestrogen therapy with regard to cardiovascular changes have to be weighed against their benefit.

Some new epidemiological data on CHD have been provided from three different sets of population statistics. These are:

(a) the annual reports of the Austrian Ministry of Health from 1962 to 1973;
(b) a local preventive programme running for 10 years in a western district of Austria covering a population of approximately 28 000 subjects of both sexes;
(c) data collected by a multicentre trial, co-ordinated by the

63

World Health Organization, which registered cases of ischaemic heart disease during 1971 and 1972 in 18 European centres covering a population of approximately 3.5 million people.

There are several inherent difficulties in reporting the epidemiological results about the evident lower risk in women of CHD. The greatest difficulty is the low incidence rate of CHD in all female age groups. This makes statistical testing rather difficult.

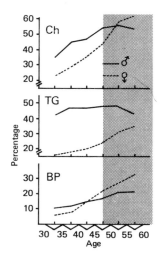

**Figure 6.8** Percentages of men and women of various ages in whom the risk factors for CHD: high plasma cholesterol, high triglyceride levels and elevated blood pressure were found

From the Austrian health statistics one can conclude that in Austria the widespread use of oral contraceptives (25–30% of all fertile women use them) did not change the cardiovascular mortality rate in any of the 5-year age groups of women between 30 and 40 years. This is at least true for the period of observation, 1962–1973 (Figure 6.7). Apparently, an increased risk of myocardial infarction in contraceptive users can only be found in women who already have a high risk for CHD.

In the health screening programme in a western part of Austria covering a population sample of approximately 10 000 women, remarkable differences in the incidence of age-dependent risk factors for CHD were found. The risk factors such as high cholesterol and triglycerides blood levels, and elevated blood pressure increase in women with age. There is a slightly steeper increase in the peri-menopausal period. This increase is most pronounced for cholesterol (Figure 6.8).

The data collected in 18 European countries during 1971 and 1972 show that the incidence of cardiovascular disease varies from one country to another. This is most evident for patients in the age groups between 40 and 55. The overall incidence rate is high in northern Europe where it is also earlier and more pronounced in pre-menopausal women (Figure 6.9). Possible factors that influence the peculiar geographic distribution of CHD might support the early increase of CHD in younger women.

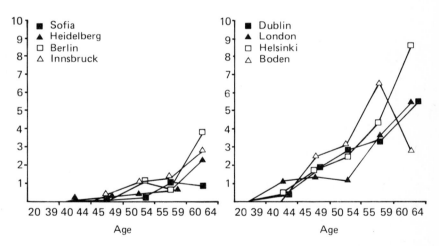

**Figure 6.9** Incidence of cardiovascular disease at various ages in several European cities

It was concluded that the incidence of coronary heart disease in the pre- and post-menopause is still a matter for debate and more investigations are needed before therapeutic consequences can be made. A potential risk of oestrogens is not likely because oral contraceptives *per se* are apparently not a risk factor for coronary heart disease.

## POST-MENOPAUSAL OSTEOPOROSIS (Introduced by G. S. Gordan)

Bone mass measurements published in the last 4 years show conclusively that loss of ovarian function by the menopause or oophorectomy causes loss of bone. Insufficient bone mass leads to increased porosity and brittleness, and a rarefaction of normally mineralized bone, which ultimately results in pathological fracture of the skeleton. Physiological bone loss occurs in both sexes, but later and to a much smaller degree in males than in females. Osteoporotic fractures due to the pathological state of osteoporosis is rarely observed in males before the age of 70. Ethnic factors are also of importance for the development of osteoporosis; in black women osteoporosis and fractures are rare. Post-menopausal osteoporosis results from a precipitous increase in bone tissue destruction when oestrogenic restraint on bone breakdown is lost. After oophorectomy trabecular bone is preferentially lost in the three sites where post-menopausal women sustain fractures: the vertebrae, wrists and hips. Some 26% of white women have osteoporotic vertebral fractures by the age of 60 and 50% by the age of 75. These cause considerable discomfort and deformity. Hip fractures entail a considerable morbidity and mortality. Hence, post-menopausal osteoporosis constitutes a major health problem for elderly white women.

This bone loss and its sequelae such as pain and deformity can be prevented by surprisingly small doses of oestrogens. Effective prophylactic doses include mestranol 20 $\mu$g, ethinyl oestradiol 20 $\mu$g or conjugated natural oestrogens 0.6 mg daily for 20–25 consecutive days each month. In far advanced pathological post-menopausal osteoporosis with fractures, therapy with full replacement doses of oestrogens can prevent further fractures. These doses include stilboestrol 1 mg, ethinyloestradiol 50 $\mu$g, methallenoestrol 6 mg or conjugated natural oestrogens 1.25 mg daily. Unlike prophylactic small doses, these frequently cause endometrial hyperplasia and bleeding. All oestrogen preparations should always be given cyclically omitting 5–10 days each month, with or without progestogen. Any break-through bleeding while taking oestrogens, i.e. any 'bleeding-not-according-to-plan' requires histological examination of the endometrium. Invasive cancers and metastases in women so treated need not occur. Deaths from this cause are very rare, while female deaths from preventible osteoporotic hip fracture are frequent.

Whether other oestrogenic preparations are equally suitable for prophylactic and therapeutic use in post-menopausal osteoporosis, has to be investigated. One research preparation, viz. OD 14, an oestrogenic anabolic steroid, seems very promising.

## SUMMARY

It is impossible to summarize the great amount of data presented and discussed, and all the well-considered suggestions made in the course of this workshop. One thing, however, became very clear indeed: the menopause and the post-menopausal life-span, though physiological events, can be responsible for a considerable number of disturbances which do react impressively to therapy, particularly to sex hormone supplementation. It also emerged indisputably that knowledge is growing fast regarding the use of effective doses of sex hormones which bear little risk of causing iatrogenic harm to the patient.

# Oestrogen and progesterone receptors

## Moderator: A. M. Kaye

Department of Hormone Research, The Weizmann Institute of Science, Rehovoth, Israel


*Participants invited to present their views at this workshop included:*

*H. Jacobson (USA)*
*P. W. Jungblut (West Germany)*
*R. J. B. King (United Kingdom)*
*G. A. Puca (Italy)*

According to current views, steroid hormones function by binding to specific receptor proteins present in responsive cells. Although a general scheme of steroid interaction with the cell has been elucidated, the precise mechanism by which steroids enhance RNA and protein synthesis is still unknown. One central approach to the problem of understanding the mechanism of oestrogen action is by isolating, purifying and characterizing the various components of this mechanism and by studying the mode of interaction of these parts under simplified conditions *in vitro*, to contribute to knowledge of how the mechanism works as a whole.

Various forms of oestrogen receptors have been identified in uterine tissue: (i) the 'native' receptor, localized in the extranuclear space of the cell, which is characterized by the reversible change of its sedimentation coefficient on sucrose gradients from 8 to 4S when the salt concentration is increased from 0.1 to 0.4 M (Jensen *et al.*, 1968); (ii) the 'derived' cytosol receptor, sedimenting at 4S in low or high salt, which is obtained from the 'native' receptor on activation by a $Ca^{2+}$-dependent enzyme (Puca *et al.*, 1977); (iii) the 'nuclear' receptor, the form that migrates from the cytosol into the nucleus after formation of the hormone–receptor complex (Jensen *et al.*, 1968; Puca and Bresciani, 1968). It is possible that there is a special function for each form.

Purification of the various forms of oestradiol receptor is a very difficult task because of their scarcity in biological tissues: in the uterus, where they reach the highest concentration, it can be estimated that there is about half a milligram of receptor protein per kilogram of tissue. Although the 'derived' form of receptor could be purified by affinity chromatography on oestradiol adsorbents (Sica *et al.*, 1973), the 'native' oestradiol receptor resisted all attempts at purification because of its tendency to form large and irreversible aggregates.

## PURIFICATION OF THE NATIVE FORM OF THE OESTRADIOL RECEPTOR OF CALF UTERUS

Recently Molinari *et al.* (1977) described a property which is peculiar to the 'native' form of the oestradiol receptor, its ability to interact specifically with heparin bound covalently to Sepharose. This property permitted the purification of this form of the receptor to apparent homogeneity.

Oestradiol–receptor complexes interact with heparin–agarose with a very high affinity. Cations increase the association constant of the interaction approximately 10-fold: from $5 \times 10^9$ $M^{-1}$ in 0.5 mM EDTA, to $4 \times 10^{10}$ $M^{-1}$ in 5 mM $Mg^{2+}$. Among cations tested, $Mn^{2+}$ is the most effective (maximal stimulation at 2 mM) followed by $Mg^{2+}$; but $Sr^{2+}$, $Ba^{2+}$ and $Fe^{2+}$ are also effective. Even though oestradiol is not required for the binding of the receptor on heparin–agarose columns, determination of affinity indicates an oestradiol dependence of the interaction. When the receptor is complexed with hormone, the affinity is at least 10 times higher. Elution of the bound oestradiol–receptor complex or oestradiol-free receptor from heparin–agarose is obtained by increasing the ionic strength of the buffer above 0.2 M (NaCl, KCl, KBr, NaSCN), or by adding guanidine-HCl (1 M) or heparin in solution (1 to 5 mg/ml). EDTA (up to 100 mM) or cations (1–50 mM) have no effect on elution nor do they modify the elution by heparin or salts.

Sucrose gradient analysis of uterine cytosol before and after contact with heparin–agarose shows that 'native' 8S receptor disappears after incubation of the crude cytosol with heparin–agarose (Molinari *et al.*, 1977). Transformation of 'native' receptors by the $Ca^{2+}$-dependent receptor transforming factor (RTF) (Puca *et al.*, 1968) causes the complete loss of this property (Molinari *et al.*, 1977).

Nuclear receptor, obtained from rats after *in vivo* injection of physiological doses of oestradiol, does not interact with heparin–agarose (Molinari *et al.*, 1977). The fact that the nuclear and the RTF-transformed receptors have both lost the binding site for

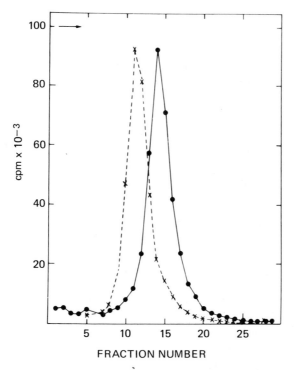

**Figure 7.1** Sucrose gradient analysis of oestradiol–receptor complex eluted from heparin–agarose. Samples of 0.3 ml were applied to 10–30% sucrose gradients in low salt buffer ( ● — ● ) or in high salt (0.4 M KCl) buffer ( × — × ); and centrifuged for 11 h at 55 000 rev/min at 2 °C using a Spinco SW-60 Ti rotor. The arrow indicates the direction of sedimentation

heparin could reflect the loss of a hypothetical binding site of the native receptor for extranuclear components. Thus, RTF might in this way permit receptor transfer from cytosol to nucleus.

The specific interaction of 'native' oestradiol–receptor with heparin–agarose can be utilized in the purification of this form. Puca then presented a simplified purification procedure.

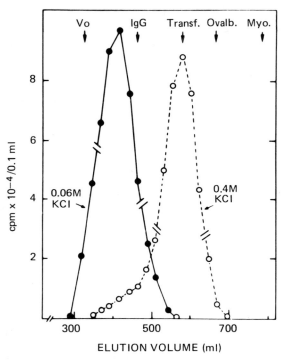

**Figure 7.2** Chromatography of oestradiol–receptor complex, eluted from heparin–agarose, on Sephadex G-200 columns equilibrated in low (0.06 M KCl) salt ( ● — ● ) and in high (0.4 M KCl) salt ( o — o ) buffer. The column (total volume = 962 ml) was developed with an *upward flow* of 30 ml/h and was partially equilibrated with heparin (0.1 mg/ml) before the application of the sample. $V_0$ indicates peak elution of blue dextran

[$^3$H]oestradiol labelled cytosol is incubated batchwise for 1 h at 0 °C with an amount of heparin–agarose able to immobilize 80–90% of the oestradiol receptor complex (usually from 5 to 10 g of packed heparin–agarose in 100 ml of cytosol). It is recommended to fractionate the cytosol in portions of this size in order to use the minimal amount of resin and obtain the advantages of a small elution volume as well as a better purification. The gel is then packed in a column, washed with buffer containing 0.18 M KCl and then eluted with a buffer containing 3 mg/ml of heparin. Recovery is usually greater than 50% of the oestradiol–receptor complex originally present in the crude cytosol, and purification factors vary between 50- and 350-fold. The simplified purification procedure is based on the salt dissociation property of the 'native' receptor. The [$^3$H]oestradiol–receptor complex eluted from heparin–agarose sediments at 6S in low ionic strength buffer while in buffer containing 0.4 M KCl it sediments as a sharp peak at 4S (Figure 7.1). Similarly on Sephadex G-200 columns (Figure 7.2) equilibrated in low salt,

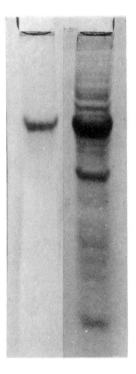

**Figure 7.3** Electrophoresis of oestradiol receptor on polyacrylamide slab gel in 0.1% sodium dodecyl sulphate. Protein samples are mixed with equal volumes of 30 mM sodium phosphate buffer, pH 7, 2% $\beta$-mercaptoethanol, 2% sodium dodecyl sulphate and incubated at 37 °C for 2 h. A single receptor protein band is observed of slightly lower mobility than the albumin component of the cytosol, run in the other well

the complex elutes between the void volume of the column and immunoglobulin, with an apparent molecular weight of about 300 000. When the salt concentration of the column buffer is brought to 0.4 M KCl, the complex elutes with a molecular weight of about 70 000. If the oestradiol–receptor complex eluted from heparin–agarose is first chromatographed on a Sephadex G-200 column equilibrated in low salt and then, after concentration, it is applied to a second Sephadex G-200 column equilibrated in 0.4 M KCl, a fast and simple purification is achieved.

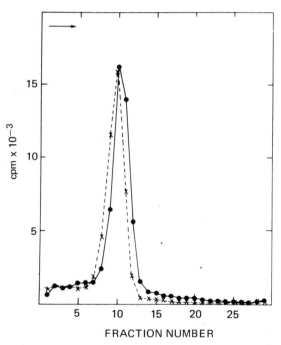

**Figure 7.4** Sucrose gradient analysis of purified oestradiol–receptor complex in low salt ( ● — ● ) or in high (0.4 M KCl) salt ( × — × ). Conditions are identical to those described in the legend to Figure 7.1

The purified receptor shows a single band of protein of 69 000 molecular weight on sodium dodecyl sulphate polyacrylamide gel electrophoresis (Figure 7.3). By sucrose gradient analysis it sediments at 4.3S in the presence or in the absence of 0.4 M KCl (Figure 7.4). Pure 'native' receptor still maintains its high tendency to aggregate. In fact, it does not penetrate into the polyacrylamide gel in non-dissociating conditions and elutes in the void volumes of Sephadex G-200 columns equilibrated in low salt buffer. Small concentrations of heparin (0.01%) are required to maintain the 'native' receptor in the non-aggregated form.

Availability of pure receptor opens the way to further biochemical characterization and investigation of the role of this important protein in the control of gene expression.

## TURNOVER OF RECEPTORS

Receptors for oestradiol are found in (i) the cytosol, (ii) the microsomes, and (iii) the nuclei of target organs. They all contain the same binding site, but differ in extractability, net charge and – depending on their functional state – in sedimentation velocity (Little et al., 1975; Jungblut et al., 1976). The study of their interrelationship by depletion/replenishment experiments requires a quantitative extraction. This is difficult to achieve with fresh uteri. Jungblut reported on investigations on whether the various receptors can be sequentially extracted from disrupted frozen cells in spite of the fragmentation of subcellular structures caused by the homogenization procedure.

Results indicated that the 'acidic' cytosol receptor is easily extracted, the 'basic' microsomal receptor is membrane-bound and 'acidic' nuclear receptor can be distinguished from the cytosol receptor by its poorer extractability (Jungblut, 1978).

Expressed in binding sites per cell ($7.5 \times 10^{-12}$ g DNA), the mean values were: for cytosol receptor, 8650; for 'basic' microsomal receptor, 6510 and for nuclear receptor, 3200; in total 18 400. These figures cannot be considered as constant numbers since they are subject to steroid-dependent – even in ovariectomized animals (Hughes et al., 1976) – and steroid-independent receptor turnover (Jungblut et al., 1977). The high proportion of 'basic' microsomal receptor (Little et al., 1972) emphasizes its hitherto overlooked biological significance.

Parallel studies on receptor concentration in uterine nuclei from ovariectomized and ovariectomized/adrenalectomized pigs were made using a different technique for fresh nuclei (Jungblut et al., 1978). According to the generally accepted view, oestradiol binds to an 'acidic' receptor in the cytosol, the complex immediately dimerizes and is then quickly translocated into the nucleus (Jungblut *et al.*, 1976). This concept implies that neither oestradiol nor the receptor can be concentrated in the nucleus independently. Uterine nuclei from ovariectomized animals, therefore, should contain only small amounts of oestradiol (of adrenal origin) together with a corresponding concentration of receptor, while uterine nuclei from ovariectomized/adrenalectomized animals should be devoid of both. Ovariectomized and ovariectomized/adrenalectomized pigs of the German Landrace breed were used.

The nuclear receptor extracted at 0 °C, sedimented in two peaks (4 and 5S) but in a single 5S peak when extracted at 30 °C. The 5S peak was dissociated to the 4S monomer by proton addition (pH 6.5).

**Table 7.1  Receptor and oestradiol content of pig uterus nuclei**

| Ablative treatment | Days p.o. | Binding sites per nucleus | Molecules oestradiol per nucleus |
|---|---|---|---|
| Ovariectomy | 47 | 2690 | 1480 |
| Ovariectomy | 56 | 3010 | 1270 |
| Ovariectomy | 63 | 2910 | 1210 |
| Ovariectomy | 47 | 2170 | 210 |
| Ovariectomy | 53 | 2230 | 600 |
| Ovariectomy/adrenalectomy* | 33 | 2480 | 480 |
| Ovariectomy/adrenalectomy | 33 | 2230 | 0 |
| Ovariectomy/adrenalectomy | 33 | 1230 | 0 |
| Ovariectomy/adrenalectomy | 12 | 1180 | 0 |
| Ovariectomy/adrenalectomy | 12 | 1030 | 0 |
| Ovariectomy/adrenalectomy | 10 | 1430 | 0 |
| Ovariectomy/adrenalectomy | 10 | 1180 | 0 |

\* Hypertrophied remnants of adrenal cortex found
Detection limit for binding sites and oestradiol: 60/nucleus; interassay variation: 6%

Uterine nuclei from ovariectomized animals contained more binding sites than oestradiol (Table 7.1); receptor only was found in nuclei from ovariectomized/adrenalectomized animals. Receptor thus may be translocated and dimerized in the absence of oestradiol and – judged from the fluctuations observed in ovariectomized/ hypophysectomized rats (Hughes *et al.*, 1976) – act as a transcription-regulating protein in its own right.

Whether or not there is a similar situation in humans remains to be investigated.

The oestradiol receptor content of breast cancer specimens is now widely used as an indicator for hormone sensitivity which is a prerequisite for endocrine therapy.

Recently, ovarian-independent fluctuations were described for several mammalian tissues (Hughes *et al.*, 1976) including human breast cancer:

(1) An apparent circadian rhythm influences the uterine oestrogen receptor concentration of ovariectomized rats.

(2) A seasonal variation was found in uteri of immature calves and ovariectomized pigs (Figure 7.5) and in breast cancer biopsies from post-menopausal women (see below).

(3) A fluctuation with a periodicity of 9–12 days was observed in the uteri of ovariectomized/hypophysectomized rats.

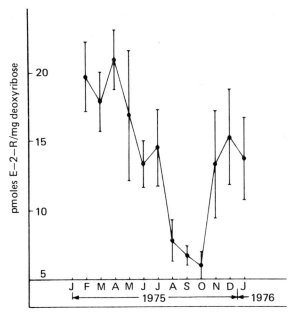

**Figure 7.5** Fluctuation in uterine oestradiol receptor (E-2-R) content of ovariectomized pigs during 12 consecutive months. Each point represents the average ± SD of 10 pools of three control horns

The absence of 'normal base-line' values considerably reduces the value of quantitative oestrogen receptor assay as the sole indicator for hormone-sensitivity. Therefore, this assay should be complemented by further criteria. The assessment of nuclear-bound oestradiol is both a logical choice and an easy task. Presence of the hormone would demonstrate that the receptor is still susceptible to steroid-facilitated conformational change, dimerization and translocation into the nucleus. Intact transcription-enhancing capability could be deduced from the presence of a specific transcription/translation product, such as the progestin receptor, the synthesis of which apparently depends on oestrogen receptor action (Horwitz and McGuire, 1975).

Together, these three parameters provide a reliable indication for hormone sensitivity, as demonstrated in a recent study by the presence, in 10 normal human uteri, of substantial amounts of oestrogen receptor, oestradiol in the nuclear fraction and progestin receptor (Jungblut *et al.*, 1977).

In mammary cancers, diverse patterns were observed: three out of 35 cancers contained neither receptor nor nuclear oestradiol. Six carcinomas contained oestrogen receptor and oestradiol in the nuclear fraction but no progestin receptor, pointing to a failure in the transcription-enhancing events. Two cancers contained no oestrogen receptor, but both nuclear oestradiol and progestin receptor were present. This could be due either to experimental error, or to the presence of undetectably small amounts of oestradiol receptor, and underlines the importance of having more than one parameter for assessing hormone sensitivity. The remaining 24 cancers showed a pattern similar to that seen in normal human uterus.

Most of the post-menopausal cancers examined contained surprisingly high nuclear oestradiol concentrations. Since oestrogen production in the ovaries declines rapidly after menopause, this oestradiol must originate from peripherally aromatized adrenal precursors. An ablative endocrine treatment of patients, whose mammary cancers fulfil all three criteria for hormone sensitivity, should therefore ideally comprise ovariectomy and adrenalectomy.

However, in view of the results reported above on uterine nuclei of pigs, it must be questioned whether even the complete withdrawal of hormones is fully effective. The higher content of receptor than oestradiol in pig nuclei could be explained either by a separate release of oestradiol and receptor which had originally entered the nucleus jointly, or by a steroid-independent entrance of the 'receptor' which in itself possesses transcription-enhancing activity. The latter possibility seems the more probable one to Jungblut – consequently receptor-'poisoning' in addition to hormone withdrawal is proposed as a therapeutic requirement. The experiments of Lippman *et al.* (1976) on human mammary cancer cell lines, the growth rates of which are enhanced by oestradiol and decreased by antioestrogens, was cited in support of this concept.

King pointed out that rodent experiments have clearly shown that nearly all of the intranuclear oestrogen receptor is complexed with oestrogen. This means that very little nuclear receptor can be detected in assays carried out at 0–4 °C. If the temperature is raised so that exchange of endogenous and exogenous oestradiol takes place, nuclear receptor can be found in oestrogen-primed animals.

In endometria from post-menopausal women receiving oestrogen therapy, the results are different. Regardless of whether the patients were receiving oestrone or oestradiol preparations, the amount of nuclear receptor assayed at 4 °C was approximately similar to the values obtained at 30 °C. The reason for the discrepancy between the rodent and human results could provide important clues as to the function of nuclear receptor. The possibility that in human endometrium there are large numbers of unoccupied nuclear receptor sites is unlikely in King's opinion: there is sufficient oestradiol present to account for all of the receptor.

## THE USE OF PROGESTERONE RECEPTOR TO DETERMINE SENSITIVITY TO OESTROGEN

It has been suggested that a change in endometrial sensitivity might occur at some stage in the events occurring in the evolution of a neoplasm. However, proof of such a change has been lacking. The experiments of King and Whitehead (1978) on the biochemistry of normal and abnormal endometria from post-menopausal women receiving oestrogen replacement therapy have provided a supply of tissue that can be used to study putative changes in endometrial sensitivity. A limited number of results indicate that an increase in endometrial sensitivity to oestrogen occurs at the stage of atypical hyperplasia. Based on these and other results, King presented a model whereby such a change in sensitivity could result in the production of a carcinoma (Figure 7.6). In essence, the model suggests that prolonged oestrogen exposure of normal endometrium leads to a relatively refractory state. Evidence for such an idea has been obtained from studies in monkeys (Hisaw and Hisaw, 1961), mice (Lee, 1972) and rats (Katzenellenbogen and Ferguson, 1975; Lobl and Maenza, 1975; Stormshak *et al.*, 1976). During the transition from normal to one of the hyperplastic conditions, this refractoriness is lost, resulting in a prolonged, elevated oestrogen sensitivity. Such a change, if translated into an increased cell proliferation rate, would allow the differential development of abnormal relative to normal cells. Subsequent appearance of a carcinoma would be accompanied by the formation of cells of variable sensitivities that characterize such tumours.

The idea of a refractory state under the influence of prolonged oestrogen treatment was suggested to King by the results presented in the references quoted above and by assay of nuclear oestrogen receptor and soluble progesterone receptor in post-menopausal endometria (King *et al.*, 1978). It was noticed that after 2 weeks of oestrogen treatment (either derivatives of oestrone or oestradiol) oestrogen receptor levels reached a maximum of about 8000 molecules/cell nucleus and by the third week had fallen to about 5000 molecules/nucleus. This fall could be interpreted as a decline in endometrial sensitivity to oestrogen and, as it was not accompanied by a change in the proportion of total cellular receptor in the nucleus, suggested a fall in efficiency of the overall oestrogen receptor machinery. It was further observed that progesterone receptor was positively correlated with oestrogen receptor in pre-menopausal endometria but a negative correlation existed in post-menopausal endometria obtained during the third week of oestrogen treatment.

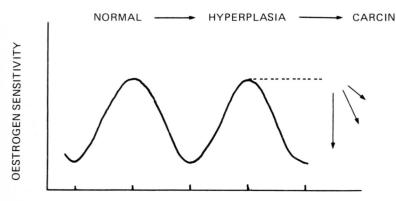

**Figure 7.6** Model for changes in endometrial sensitivity to oestrogen leading to the development of carcinoma

The amount of progesterone receptor can be used as an index of oestrogenic activity (as mentioned above); hence the post-menopausal results indicate a refractoriness that is not apparent in the pre-menopausal samples.

If there is a change in oestrogen sensitivity, it should exhibit itself as abnormal proportions of progesterone receptor to oestrogen receptor. No such change was detected in comparing endometria histologically normal except for hyperplasia; but an approximately two-fold increase in the ratio between progesterone and oestrogen receptors existed between normal and atypical hyperplasia. This difference was not seen in specimens that had normal histology at the time of assay but which had come from women who had previously presented with atypical hyperplasia. The change in the progesterone to oestrogen receptor ratio was mainly due to elevated progesterone receptor levels.

It should be stressed that the proposed model is based on sparse evidence but it does suggest a different line of experimentation to that adopted in most experiments aimed at elucidating the mechanism of oestrogen action. The majority of such experiments are of the acute type in which biochemical changes are observed for a short time after one or two oestrogen injections; chronic treatment of much longer duration might yield different results to those obtained with acute experiments and provide data to determine the validity of the model.

Schwarz (Utrecht) pointed out that such a diminished response to oestrogen might be an explanation for the clinical fact that women treated for mammary cancer with massive doses of oestradiol do not show withdrawal bleeding at cessation of therapy.

Jacobson commented that in experiments in which he administered oestrogen plus progestin to monkeys over a long period, the group receiving the highest dose showed no oestradiol uptake in the uterus at the end of the experiment.

## RECEPTORS IN THE MENOPAUSE: AGE-RELATED CHANGES IN THE CONCENTRATION OF CYTOPLASMIC OESTROGEN RECEPTORS IN HUMAN TISSUES

Although the principal receptor-containing organ of interest to this workshop is the uterus, an oestrogen target organ in which changes in receptor concentration could after uterine function or sensitivity

81

in ways that might well be apparent to the gynaecologist, we would also be interested in analogous receptor changes in hypothalamus, pituitary or ovary. These changes could alter the oestrogen-modulated secretory activities of these organs.

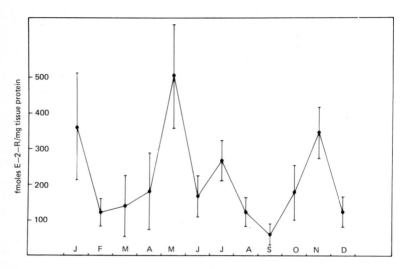

**Figure 7.7** Fluctuation in the mean monthly values ± SD of oestradiol receptor (E-2-R) content in primary mammary cancers of post-menopausal women. Graph based on 84 receptor-positive specimens collected in 5½ years. Number of cases per calendar months January–December were 3, 8, 8, 7, 8, 5, 8, 8, 5, 9, 9 and 6, respectively

Prospective studies to investigate such phenomena in women range from difficult to impossible; in animals we cannot study an ovarian menopause. Jacobson and his colleagues therefore proceeded to examine concentration/age relationships in another human organ, the receptor-containing adenocarcinoma of the mammary gland. They are now rapidly accumulating such data as tumour specimens are analysed to provide physicians with diagnostic information. They make the reasonable assumption that if receptor concentrations are altered in normal organs by exposure to some humoral agent, a similar regulation would be manifest in all receptor-containing cells of the individual, including cancer cells to which she is host.

If one proposes that there is in mammary tumours a concentration of cytoplasmic oestrogen receptor that is related to the age of the patient, it must, as has recently been shown, be interpreted with relation to the season of the year (Jungblut, 1978). The concentration of oestrogen receptor in mammary tumour specimens is *seasonal* (Figure 7.7) with a maximum in May, a minimum in September, and a maximum/minimum ratio of approximately 10 : 1. Statistical analysis indicated this is not likely to have occurred by chance. Subsequently similar seasonality has been seen in five other data sets: Rdam, Ben May 1974, Ben May 1975, Albany and Nijmegen. It is exceedingly difficult to prove seasonality; it probably cannot be done with any of these five individually.

Another practical approach is to call the first set the *Index* set. Note that the maximum is in the second calendar quarter, and the minimum is in the third. Therefore, if quarterly means for the oestrogen receptor in the Wilhelmshaven series of tumours is calculated, the direction of change is shown by the arrows as follows: I ↑ II ↓ III ↑ IV. Comparing the five others to the Wilhelmshaven, there are $5 \times 3 = 15$ arrows; 14 were found to agree with the index. The probability of this occurring by chance is very low –

$$p = \frac{15}{2^{15}} = \frac{15}{32768} = 0.00046$$

This phenomenon is relevant to uterine biology. In the ovariectomized pig the concentrations of receptors were found to be seasonal: a maximum in the spring, a minimum in the autumn, with a maximum/minimum ratio of roughly 5 (Figure 7.5).

This phenomenon is also relevant to *organ responsiveness to oestrogens*. Using the New York State Department of Health Cancer Registry data, the frequency of reports of breast cancer was shown to be maximal in May and minimal in August. This observation fits the hypothesis that oestrogen dependent breast tumours following the seasonal oestrogen receptor pattern, would be most sensitive to oestrogen and would grow fastest in May. Women would become aware of breast masses with greater frequency in that month. Since the interval between mass discovery and histological confirmation of diagnosis is usually short, the result found could be anticipated.

The pituitary gland also shows seasonal variations in oestrogen receptor concentration. The ovariectomized ewe has high plasma levels of LH that can be suppressed by injection of oestrogen, but only if the oestrogen is given during the season when ewes are in anoestrous. The pituitary concentration of oestrogen receptor is seasonal in the ewe, being highest in the anoestrous months.

## Seasonal sensitivity to oestrogen of the human pituitary

A Japanese report described seasonality in the rate of conceptions of twins in that country. The pattern is bimodal, and is similar to the oestrogen receptor pattern described above, with extremes in June and October, about one month later than the oestrogen receptor extremes. Jacobson proposes that this relates to hypothalamic or pituitary sensitivity to oestrogen (i.e. oestrogen receptor concentrations) in Japanese women, modulating the cyclic LH surges and the probability of plural ovulation.

Having presented a case for the 'universality' of oestrogen receptor biorhythms, the cause must be considered.

Based on prior findings with the oestrogen receptor in the ovariectomized rat uterus, it was considered likely that seasonal variations in tissue oestrogen receptors were caused by oestrogen receptor suppression induced by hormonal substances secreted by the adrenal gland at a rate dependent upon the season. Evidence for seasonality in adrenal secreting activity was sought. A reliable published account (Halberg-Hamburger 17-ketosteroid excretion) was found. The daily 17-ketosteroids from one man were examined for 15 years, and showed a biomodal seasonal pattern with a minimum in May and a maximum in September. This is the inverse of the receptor pattern, and supports the hypothesis of receptor suppression by an adrenal product. However, the amplitude of the seasonal swings, though significant, is very low (a few per cent).

Data on etiocholanolone excretion in the urine of women with breast cancer also shows seasonality. Twenty-four-hour urine specimens obtained from 100 women just prior to adrenalectomy for advanced breast disease were analysed in a National Cancer Institute supported co-operative study, attempting to find women who had a high probability of benefiting from adrenalectomy for treatment of their disease. The daily etiocholanolone data when plotted by month of collection resembles the previous male 17-ketosteroid pattern but with a much higher amplitude ratio (maximum $\simeq 3.2$).

Etiocholanolone in the urine of more than 200 mastectomy candidates was also measured. These data showed a simple unimodal pattern with an etiocholanolone maximum appearing in the fall and a maximum/minimum ratio of 3.2.

For investigating the relationship between menopause and oestrogen receptor concentration, a group of 853 patients from whom primary cancer specimens were recovered during 1976–8 were considered. Pre-menopausal (younger) women were found to have lower oestrogen receptor concentrations but with a general trend upward with advancing age. These patients are described in Table 7.2.

**Table 7.2  Classification of patients from whom primary breast cancer specimens were recovered**

|  | Patients | Oestrogen receptor positive cancers |
|---|---|---|
| Pre-menopausal | 193 | 99 |
| Peri-menopausal | 11 | 5 |
| Post-menopausal | 649 | 433 |
| TOTAL | 853 | 537 |

The rise in concentration of oestrogen receptors with age in breast cancer, when analysed by 5-year age groups showed 'hesitation' from age 60–80, and then resumed fast upward movement. This data from Albany is parallel to data from the Ben May Laboratory which shows an upward climb of oestrogen receptor values to the 70–74-year-old age group, followed by a decline.

A personal communication from Cortez (Interlab Associates) states that a *decline* occurs at 70–80 years which is statistically significant; the rise then resumes.

Jacobson concluded that in primary breast cancer: (i) pre-menopausal oestrogen receptor concentration is less than post-menopausal, (ii) after menopause, oestrogen receptor increases with age, (iii) this phenomenon represents a continuous process independent of follicular oestrogen, (iv) there might be a singularity in the 7th decade of life that is biologically important and should be investigated, (v) by all the prior arguments, these findings also represent uterine biology. They therefore argue for increasing uterine sensitivity to oestrogen with age, which should be investigated experimentally.

Thijssen (Utrecht) commented that in the breast cancer specimens which he assayed for oestrogen receptor concentration, he did not find any seasonal variation.

In summary of the workshop, while the criteria of concentration of oestrogen and progesterone receptors should be useful in screening compounds for their diverse effects in steroid treatment, the phenomenon of 'spare receptor capacity' for oestrogen (Clark and Peck, 1976) must be considered, and the multifactored relationship between responsiveness to the steroid hormone and the concentration of its receptors (Kaye, 1978) must be borne in mind.

## References

Clark, J. H. and Peck, E. J. (1976). Nuclear retention of receptor–oestrogen complex and nuclear acceptor sites. *Nature (Lond.)*, **260**, 635

Hisaw, F. L. and Hisaw, F. L. (1961). Action of estrogen and progesterone on the reproductive tract of lower primates. In: *Sex and Internal Secretions*, 3rd edn. (W. C. Young and G. W. Corner, eds.), pp. 556–589. (Baltimore: Williams and Wilkins)

Horwitz, K. B. and McQuire, W. L. (1975). Predicting response to endocrine therapy in human breast cancer: an hypothesis. *Science*, **189**, 726

Hughes, A., Jacobson, H. I., Wagner, R. K. and Jungblut, P. W. (1976). Ovarian-independent fluctuations of estradiol receptor levels in mammalian tissues. *Mol. Cell. Endocrinol.*, **5**, 379

Jensen, E. V., Suzuki, T., Kawashima, W., Stumpf, P., Jungblut, P. W. and De Sombre, E. R. (1968). A two-step mechanism for the interaction of estradiol with rat uterus. *Proc. Nat. Acad. Sci. (Wash.)*, **59**, 632·

Jungblut, P. (1978). Sequential extraction of various forms of estradiol receptor. *Acta Endocrinol.*, **87** (Suppl. 215), 137

Jungblut, P. W., Gaues, J., Hughes, A., Kallweit, E., Sierralta, W., Szendro, P. and Wagner, R. K. (1976). Activation of transcription regulating proteins by steroids. *J. Steroid Biochem.*, **7**, 1109

Jungblut, P. W., Hughes, A., Sierralta, W. and Wagner, R. K. (1977). A proposal for assessment of hormone sensitivity and consequent endocrine therapy of breast cancer. *Eur. J. Cancer*, **13**, 1201

Jungblut, P. W., Kallweit, E., Sierralta, W., Truitt, A. J. and Wagner, R. K. (1978). Estradiol and receptor content of uterine nuclei from ovariectomized and ovariectomized/adrenalectomized pigs. *Acta Endocrinol.*, **87** (Suppl. 215), 136

Katzenellenbogen, B. S. and Ferguson, E. R. (1975). Anti-estrogen action in the uterus: biological ineffectiveness of nuclear-bound estradiol after anti-estrogen. *Endocrinology*, **97**, 1

Kaye, A. M. (1978). The ontogeny of estrogen receptors. In: *Biochemical Actions of Hormones* (G. Litwack, ed.), Vol. 5. (New York: Academic Press)

King, R. J. B., Whitehead, M., Campbell, S. and Minardi, J. (1978). Biochemical studies on endometrium from post-menopausal women receiving hormone replacement therapy. *Postgrad. Med. J.*, **54** (Suppl. 2), 65

Lee, A. E. (1972). Cell division and DNA synthesis in the mouse uterus during continuous oestrogen treatment. *J. Endocrinol.*, **55**, 507

Lippmann, M., Bolan, G., Monaco, M., Pinkus, L. and Engel, L. (1976). Model systems for the study of estrogen action in tissue culture. *J. Steroid Biochem.*, **7**, 1045

Little, M., Rosenfeld, G. C. and Jungblut, P. W. (1972). Cytoplasmic estradiol 'receptors' associated with the 'microsomal' fraction of pig uterus. *Hoppe-Seylers Z. Physiol. Chem.*, **353**, 231

Little, M., Szendro, P., Teran, C., Hughes, A. and Jungblut, P. W. (1975). Biosynthesis and transformation of microsomal and cytosol estradiol receptors. *J. Steroid Biochem.*, **6**, 493

Lobl, R. T. and Maenza, R. M. (1975). Androgenization: alterations in uterine growth and morphology. *Biol. Reprod.*, **13**, 255

Molinari, A. M., Medici, N., Moncharmont, B. and Puca, G. A. (1977). Estradiol receptor of calf uterus: interaction with heparin–agarose and purification. *Proc. Nat. Acad. Sci. (USA)*, **74**, 4886

Puca, G. A. and Bresciani, F. (1968). Receptor molecule for oestrogens from rat uterus. *Nature (Lond.)*, **218**, 134

Puca, G. A., Nola, E., Sica, V. and Bresciani, F. (1977). Estrogen binding proteins of calf uterus. *J. Biol. Chem.*, **252**, 1358

Sica, V., Parikh, I., Nola, E., Puca, G. A. and Cuatrecasas, P. (1973). Affinity chromatography and the purification of estrogen receptors. *J. Biol. Chem.*, **248**, 6543

Stormshak, F., Leake, R., Wertz, N. and Gorski, J. (1976). Stimulatory and inhibitory effects of estrogen on uterine DNA synthesis. *Endocrinology*, **99**, 1501

# Metabolic changes due to menopause and their response to oestrogen

## Moderator: W. H. Utian
Case Western Reserve University School of Medicine,
Cleveland, Ohio, USA

## Secretary: G. S. Gordan
Lady Davies Visiting Professor, Hebrew University, Jerusalem, Israel,
on leave from the University of California, San Francisco, USA

*Participants invited to present their views at this
workshop included:*

*G. S. Gordan (USA)*
*A. A. Haspels (The Netherlands)*
*H. Kopera (Austria)*
*U. Larsson-Cohn (Sweden)*
*R. Lindsay (United Kingdom)*
*M. Notelovitz (USA)*
*M. E. L. Paterson (United Kingdom)*
*G. Samsioe (Sweden)*
*R. L. Sitruk-Ware (France)*
*J. W. W. Studd (United Kingdom)*
*M. Thom (United Kingdom)*

## INTRODUCTION

A mere decade ago the following comment appeared in a review of
the current status of menopause and oestrogen research:

'Most of what is published is based on emotional and philosophical premises; the change of life is an emotional subject not only to women, but to men and doctors.' (Utian, 1968).

From then on there developed an ever-escalating volume of research, some outstandingly good and some open to severe criticism for lack of scientific foundation. The point in time has now been reached when the individual scientist has to be content to merely maintain his research activities in a specific area of climacteric research, rather than attempt to cover the entire field. This is reflected in the ever-expanding medical literature, fully reviewed elsewhere (Utian, 1977).

Fortunately, a number of excellent workshops on oestrogens and on the menopause have been organized in recent years (van Keep and Lauritzen, 1973 and 1975; Lauritzen and van Keep, 1978), and there was also the First International Congress on the Menopause, which was held in France in 1976 (van Keep et al., 1976). These meetings have given involved researchers the opportunity to correlate efforts, to prevent excessive duplication, and to highlight areas in which information is lacking.

The purpose of this 'metabolic' workshop was to evaluate the progress that has been achieved since the 1976 meeting, and to clarify some problems deserving further efforts. Four areas were considered:

– Bone metabolism;
– Lipid metabolism;
– Carbohydrate metabolism;
– Tryptophan and vitamin $B_6$ metabolism.

The importance of this workshop cannot be over-emphasized. There is an urgent need for a consensus of opinion as to which metabolic effects of the climacteric and of oestrogen replacement therapy carry benefit, and which carry risk, so that the risk : benefit ratio can be precisely calculated.

## BONE METABOLISM

### Background

The subject of oestrogens and bones was dealt with in depth at the First International Congress on the Menopause (van Keep et al.,

1976). There was general agreement at that meeting, as indeed there is in the literature (Utian, 1977), that menopause, premature or otherwise, is associated with a negative calcium balance, increased bone resorption, and the development of osteoporosis with subsequent increased risk of bone fracture.

It was also felt at that meeting that oestrogen therapy delays or prevents loss of bone in post-menopausal women, and may even increase it, but there was disagreement as to the mechanism, that is to say, the way in which loss of oestrogen causes bone resorption. The following mechanisms were considered possible:

(1) An anticatabolic effect of oestrogens on collagenous tissues in general.
(2) An undue sensitivity of bone to the action of parathyroid hormones in the absence of oestrogens.
(3) An altered sensitivity of bone to growth hormone or to thyroid hormone.
(4) An actual deficiency of growth hormone.
(5) A deficiency of calcitonin.

As already mentioned, the purpose of the present workshop was not to re-trace the efforts of the previous meeting, but to evaluate the information which has become available since that time.

## Workshop presentations and discussion

### Prevention and treatment of post-menopausal osteoporosis (Introduced by G. S. Gordan and R. Lindsay)

Post-menopausal bone loss occurs in almost all women. Pathological bone loss with fractures causes much morbidity and mortality in non-black women after the age of 60 and constitutes an ever-increasing public health problem. This bone loss can be prevented by (1) low-dose oestrogen replacement, (2) high-dose oral calcium therapy, or (3) low-dose calcitonin therapy. Once fractures have occurred only full replacement doses of oestrogens have so far been shown to prevent further fractures. Metabolically, surprisingly small doses of oestrogens inhibit bone resorption. Since formation and resorption are necessarily linked, there is also a homeostatic decrease in bone formation. The net effect is an increase in bone mass, despite a slight rise in parathyroid hormone levels. Oral calcium carbonate in large doses also prevents post-menopausal bone loss. Since parathyroid hormone levels decrease, a slight rise in serum calcium is likely. Calcitonin directly inhibits bone resorption. Why black women are protected from osteoporosis and fractures remains to be elucidated (Gordan and Vaughn, 1977).

The most important information on efficacy of various proposed treatments for post-menopausal bone loss comes from very recent methods for measuring bone mass. The earliest, by Meema and Meema, using X-ray densitometry with a step-wedge reference, showed that at all ages men have more bone than women. Age-related bone loss is very different in the two sexes, being earlier, more rapid, and proceeding to a much greater degree in women than in men (50% versus 25%). Women lose no bone until the menopause or oophorectomy. They then lose 1–2% per year, possibly more rapidly in the first 6 years, then at a slower but continual rate. Similar data have been obtained by photon absorptiometry (Lindsay et al., 1976).

Osteodensitometry and photon absorptiometry yield similarly highly precise data in experienced hands, but positioning is a serious problem with some commercial instruments. Cortical thickness measuring, the cheapest method generally available, correlates well with both methods.

Exciting new developments for measuring vertebral spongiosa are dual-beam X-ray spectrophotometry (Dalén et al., 1974) and computed tomography and other new techniques are also under study.

When investigating the minimal osteotrophic effect of conjugated oestrogens administered in a double-blind study to oophorectomized women, Gordan found that computed tomography showed loss of vertebral spongiosa before any change was detected by cortical thickness measuring or by photon absorptiometry. Thus women at greatest risk of early osteoporosis can be investigated by this means before pathological fractures of osteoporosis occur.

Lindsay presented data that post-oophorectomy bone loss occurs at a rate inversely proportional to the blood oestrone + oestradiol level. He found that in placebo matched patients bone loss occurred more rapidly in the first 4 years post-castration ($2\frac{1}{2}$% per year) and then at a slower rate (1% per year). Cortical thickness measuring and photon absorptiometry yielded similar data.

Recker and his co-workers, who found that all three methods gave similar results, found that post-menopausal bone loss could be prevented by giving 0.6 mg conjugated oestrogens and 5 mg methyl testosterone daily, and that the results with 2.6 g calcium carbonate daily were almost as good (Recker *et al.*, 1977).

The steroid tibolone (OD 14, Organon) protects against bone loss in doses which do not stimulate the endometrium. A progestational compound, gestronol, also protects the skeleton, as does 0.3 mg conjugated oestrogens daily. Oestriol, however, in doses up to 8 mg per day has been found to be ineffective (Lindsay *et al.*, 1978).

Women with high urinary cortisol excretion lose bone most rapidly.

The consensus of opinion at this workshop was that bone biopsy was inappropriate for routine use. Fluoride and vitamin D therapy were considered toxic and probably ineffective for the treatment of post-menopausal osteoporosis.

## Summary and conclusions

New and more appropriate methods for measuring bone density have allowed long-term prospective evaluations of the effect on bone of ovarian function and post-menopausal hormone replacement therapy. The results confirm the existence of post-menopausal osteoporosis as a real entity. Furthermore, long-term low-dose oestrogen replacement is effective in preventing such bone loss. The few existing prospective studies indicate that this skeletal protective effect probably results in a reduction in bone fracture rates, but a definitive prospective controlled study is needed in order that this expectation may be confirmed. The selection of oestrogen is of importance, and several current studies should provide more definitive data in this respect.

## LIPID METABOLISM

### Background

Castration and the normal climacteric appear to be related to change in the blood lipid profile, the development of atheromatosis, and an increase in hypertension, and in the incidence of clinical coronary heart disease. The relationship appears to be indirect, however, and there is no uniform agreement about it (Utian, 1971; Blanc *et al.*, 1977; Heller and Jacobs, 1978). The initial optimism that oestrogen replacement therapy would prevent coronary heart disease has, however, taken an about turn, and the question now being asked is: Does oestrogen therapy constitute a risk factor for the development of coronary heart disease?

Cardiovascular changes in premature menopause may be important. Oophorectomy before the age of 30 has been reported to be associated with an increase in cholesterol, triglycerides, and a significant increase in the incidence of coronary vascular disease (Johansson et al., 1975). On the other hand, oestrogen replacement does not significantly reduce plasma cholesterol, in itself an accepted coronary risk factor (Utian, 1972). This finding has been confirmed, and triglyceride levels have been found to be essentially unchanged in patients treated with oestradiol and oestriol (Walters and Jensen, 1977). Nor is there any evidence of a statistically significant association between current regular use of oestrogens and the incidence of non-fatal acute myocardial infarction (Rosenberg et al., 1976).

The consensus of opinion at the First International Congress on the Menopause was that, judging from the limited data available, it seems that post-menopausal oestrogen replacement therapy does not induce changes in the plasma lipids that could be considered alarming (van Keep et al., 1976). There is urgent need, however, for more well-controlled studies of the influence of various types of oestrogen in different dose levels on post-menopausal lipid and lipoprotein metabolism.

## Workshop presentations and discussions

### Effects of natural and of synthetic oestrogens on lipoprotein fractions (Introduced by U. Larsson-Cohn)

Numerous epidemiological and experimental studies have established that increased VLDL (very low density lipoprotein) and/or LDL (low density lipoprotein) concentrations are related to an increased risk of ischaemic cardiovascular disease, while HDL (high density lipoprotein) seems to have the opposite effect.

In a recent study 6 months of post-menopausal treatment with 2 mg oestradiol valerianate raised HDL 10–15% and had little effect on other lipoprotein fractions. When 0.05 mg ethinyl oestradiol was given HDL and triglyceride (e.g. mainly VLDL) concentrations increased 30–40%. It is concluded that the long-term consequences of oestrogens on lipid and lipoprotein metabolism are complex and incompletely understood at the present time.

### Serum lipids and lipoproteins in bilaterally oophorectomized and hysterectomized women (Introduced by G. Samsioe)

Thirteen young women with histories of cervical carcinoma stage IB, for which they had undergone Wertheim–Meigs operations at least 5 years earlier but who were apparently healthy with no signs of recurrence of the disease, were put on various orally administered hormonal replacement regimens for 6-week periods. Each 6-week period was followed by a 6-week 'wash-out' period.

A dose of 20 μg ethinyl oestradiol daily led to an increase in serum triglycerides and phospholipids, while total cholesterol remained fairly unchanged. The addition of 10 mg norethisterone increased this derangement even further, and led to an 'atherogenic pattern', i.e. an increased LDL fraction with huge amounts of cholesterol ester in it, and a decrease of the HDL fraction.

A totally different pattern was found when 2 mg oestradiol valerianate was administered daily. There was a decrease in triglycerides, and changes in the lipid distribution and absolute values of the lipoprotein fractions. The decrease in LDL and VLDL, concomitant with an increase in HDL, is an 'atherosclerosis-protective' pattern. When the oestradiol valerianate dose was increased to 4 mg daily the pattern was the same as that seen when ethinyl oestradiol was given; the changes were less marked but were of the same type in the serum lipids as well as in the serum lipoproteins.

It is now well recognized that oral contraceptives are associated with an increased risk of cardiovascular disease especially in women who smoke and in those who are over 40 years of age. High levels of cholesterol and triglycerides are known to be risk factors for cardiovascular disease, and the risk is even greater when the high serum lipids are mainly within the LDL fraction of the lipoproteins.

In general, therefore, it may be said that it appears better to use natural oestrogens, rather than synthetic ones. If, however, for one reason or another, a dose of 4 mg or more oestradiol valerianate has to be given it should be realized that the 'atherosclerosis-protective' pattern with its beneficial influence on lipids and lipoprotein, which would have been seen with a lower dose, will not develop. This is most likely due to the fact that on the first liver passage a major part of the oestradiol is converted into oestrone.

An extremely sensitive method for studying lipid and lipoprotein metabolism is the determination of the fatty acid composition of serum lecithin. In the liver, lecithin is synthesized through two main pathways. The major pathway gives palmitic acid in 1-position and linoleic or oleic acid in 2-position. This pathway is stimulated by bile acids and thus indirectly by cholestasis. The other pathway yields stearic acid in 1-position and arachidonic acid in 2-position of the lecithins. This pathway is stimulated by oestrogens. Good information can therefore be obtained from a gas chromatographic analysis of the serum lecithin fatty acids.

Only in the oestradiol experiment could a typical enhancement of the oestrogen stimulated pathway be demonstrated. It therefore seems likely that the type and the dose of oestrogen replacement therapy are of importance as far as lipid and lipoprotein metabolism is concerned. In young women the changes induced by ethinyl oestradiol + a progestogen of the 19-nortesterone series seem to be of little clinical importance. However, as more risk factors are added, e.g. obesity, hypertension, and heavy smoking, serum lipoprotein metabolism may well be of great importance for the development of cardiovascular diseases.

### Effect of mestranol/norethisterone on serum lipids (Introduced by M. E. L. Paterson)

Serum cholesterol, triglycerides, and electrophoretic strips were measured on 49 patients receiving Menophase (graded sequential mestranol/norethisterone) at 0, 2, 6, and 12 months. The serum cholesterol showed a significant fall at 2, 6, and 12 months at the 0.1% level.

Conversely, the serum triglycerides showed a significant rise at the 0.1% level at 2 months and at the 1% level after 6 and 12 months.

The number of patients with normal electrophoretic strips at the various durations of therapy was the same, but there was a significant reduction in the number of patients with type IIA and type IIB hyperlipidaemia with a corresponding increase in type IV hyper-lipidaemia. A tentative suggestion is made that this converts the lipid pattern from an atherosclerotic one to a diabetogenic one.

This feature also emerged when the patients were divided into their peri- and post-menopausal subgroups.

The serum cholesterol of patients after 12 months' treatment was similar to that of a group of 45 pre-menopausal patients who had received no treatment, but, as expected, the triglyceride levels were significantly higher.

### Effects of percutaneously administered 17β-oestradiol on triglyceride levels (Introduced by R. L. Sitruk-Ware)

The effect on plasma triglyceride levels of percutaneously adminis- tered 17β-oestradiol was investigated in 53 women aged between 45 and 70 who were being treated for post-menopausal complaints. Pretreatment plasma oestradiol levels were $20 \pm 15$ pg/ml. During the course of the treatment the plasma levels of oestradiol rose to $82 \pm 30$ pg/ml.

The plasma triglyceride levels did not increase when oestradiol was administered alone, nor when it was used in association with progestins. However, in 11 patients with high pretreatment levels of blood triglycerides, 6 months of percutaneous 17β-oestradiol administration clearly provided a significant decrease of plasma tri- glycerides from $1.65 \pm 0.32$ mmol/l to $0.97 \pm 0.16$ mmol/l ($p < 0.001$). Similar variations have been observed by others when oestradiol has been administered by routes other than the oral one. These results may be constrasted to the hypertriglyceridaemia usually observed when synthetic oestrogens are given by oral administration. On the basis of this observation, there is clearly a case for the percutaneous administration of natural oestrogens as opposed to the oral adminis- tration of synthetic oestrogens.

### Summary and conclusions

Recent information suggests that different oestrogens have different effects on blood lipids. In some instances these responses are potentially adverse, but there is promise that some beneficial changes can be induced by careful drug selection and usage in correctly evaluated patients. The route of administration may also be of importance, so that conversions of oestrogen are avoided during the first liver passage.

## CARBOHYDRATE METABOLISM

### Background

Despite an ever increasing amount of literature on the relationship between pregnancy and the oral contraceptive, on the one hand, and insulin production, carbohydrate tolerance, and diabetes mellitus on the other, there are relatively few reports on the effects of pure oestrogens on these factors in post-menopausal women.

Indeed, only brief mention was made of the subject at the First International Congress on the Menopause, when it was reported that 5 years after the menopause glucose and serum immunoreactive insulin (IRI) responses to tolbutamide were not impaired. Hence, it was concluded, the menopause does not cause a disturbance of carbohydrate metabolism in women without a predisposition to diabetes. It was further stated that 3–7 years' administration of 'natural' oestrogens in the post-menopause appeared to have no diabetogenic effect in obese or non-obese women.

### Workshop presentations and discussions

*The effect of hormonal replacement therapy on glucose tolerance in post-menopausal women (Introduced by M. Thom)*

In recent years a better understanding of the changes which occur at the time of the climacteric has led to a widespread use of oestrogen therapy in the belief that symptomatic improvement will occur together with prevention or retardation of osteoporosis. The possible adverse effects of oestrogen therapy on carbohydrate metabolism were investigated by performing oral glucose tolerance tests on 50 symptomatic post-menopausal women before and after 3 months of hormone replacement therapy. The patients were randomly allocated to one of five groups and treated with various synthetic or so-called naturally occurring oestrogens. An impairment of glucose tolerance was found in 31 of the 50 patients after 3 months of therapy. Preparations containing 100 $\mu$g ethinyl oestradiol or graduated doses of up to 50 $\mu$g mestranol produced a significant deterioration of carbohydrate tolerance. The conjugated equine oestrogen (1.25 mg daily) and oestradiol valerate (2 mg daily) treated groups did not show abnormal glucose tolerance. The decrease in glucose tolerance may be due as much to dosage levels as to any metabolic

98

characteristics of the various oestrogens prescribed (Thom *et al.*, 1977).

## *The effect of oestrogen replacement therapy on carbohydrate tolerance in menopausal women (Introduced by M. Notelovitz)*

A voluminous but contradictory literature exists concerning the effect of oestrogen replacement therapy on carbohydrate metabolism in menopausal females. The consensus of opinion seems to be that oestrogen will result in alterations in glucose tolerance (GTT) in some 40–50% of patients. Our own research has indicated that this effect is less likely and less pronounced in women taking natural oestrogens. Further, although alterations in tolerance occur within the first 3 months, continuation of therapy (for a year or more) results in stabilization and normalization of the GTT in most women, with complete reversal to normal after cessation of therapy. In some, a permanent alteration of the GTT will persist. Thus every patient needs to be assessed 6 months after starting therapy and then annually with single 2-hour post-glucose blood tests. Diabetes *per se* is not an absolute contraindication to oestrogen therapy in the peri- and post-menopause.

The disturbed GTT in post-menopausal women on oestrogens is usually not accompanied by the compensatory hyperinsulinaemia noted in younger women taking oestrogen-containing oral contra-ceptives. This is not due to a lack of insulin as intravenous tolbut-amide results in the normal release of insulin. It has been noted that the incidence of abnormal GTT in post-menopausal women on oestrogens is greater after oral than after intravenous administration. This suggests that intestinal and/or hepatic modification of the insulin release/metabolic pathways may be interfered with by oestrogen therapy. Other possibilities are oestrogen-stimulated increases in cortisol, in the growth hormone, and an ill-defined increase in peripheral resistance to insulin.

## Summary and conclusions

Correct oestrogen usage does not generally result in significant or prolonged alterations in glucose tolerance, but some idiosyncratic responses may occur, and it is therefore recommended that a 2-hour post-glucose blood level be determined annually in patients on oestrogen therapy.

FEMALE AND MALE CLIMACTERIC

## TRYPTOPHAN METABOLISM

*Oestrogens, tryptophan metabolism, and vitamin B$_6$ deficiency
(Introduced by A. A. Haspels)*

Although a considerable amount of work has been carried out on the effects of contraceptive steroids on tryptophan metabolism in pre-menopausal women, less is known of the effects of hormone replacement therapy in climacteric and post-menopausal women (Haspels *et al.*, 1978).

A relative pyridoxine deficiency was found in all of 12 women using conjugated oestrogens unopposed by progestogens. This was due to disturbed tryptophan metabolism, expressed in increased xanthurenic acid excretion ($\geqslant 60\ \mu$mol/8 h) during 8 hours following the oral administration of 2 g L-tryptophan.

The intake of oestrogens has already been found to lead to a disturbance of tryptophan metabolism and to a deficiency of vitamin B$_6$. There is now evidence that this is the case not only in women taking oestrogens in oral contraceptives but also in those taking conjugated oestrogens in connection with climacteric complaints. This disturbance is clear after 1 year of oestrogen treatment. Xanthurenic acid excretion was seen to be only slightly increased in three women who used progestogens in high dosages at the same time. The biochemical changes induced could easily be corrected by the administration of vitamin B$_6$.

This is of importance for women being treated with oestrogens for climacteric complaints, as the clinical consequences of a relative vitamin B$_6$ deficiency are depressive mood, emotional instability, irritability, fatigue, disturbances in concentration and in sleep, and loss of libido. Paradoxically, the psychic disturbances resulting from conjugated oestrogen therapy in the post-menopause may to some extent be similar to those for which oestrogen therapy is prescribed around the time of the menopause itself.

## OVERALL CONCLUSION

The explosion of new information concerning the metabolic effects of post-menopausal oestrogen replacement therapy is extremely exciting. Nonetheless, considerable gaps still exist in our knowledge, and there is little room for complacency. At the current rate of

100

progress, however, much additional information can be expected to be forthcoming soon, and complex metabolic effects should then be further clarified. Renewed interest in methods of controlling metabolic changes has already led to an improvement in the selection of the oestrogens used, of the doses given, and to patient supervision.

# References

Blanc, J. J., Boschat, J., Morin, J., Clavier, J. and Penther, P. (1977). Menopause and myocardial infarction. *Am. J. Obstet. Gynecol.*, **127**, 353

Dalén, N., Lamke, B. and Wallgren, A. (1974). Bone mineral losses in oophorectomized women. *J. Bone Jt Surg.*, **56A**, 1235

Gordan, G. S. and Vaughn, C. (1977). The role of estrogens in osteoporosis. *Geriatrics*, **32**, 42

Haspels, A. A., Coelingh Bennink, H. J. T. and Schreurs, W. H. P. (1978). Disturbance of tryptophan metabolism and its correction during estrogen treatment in post-menopausal women. *Maturitas*, **1**, 15

Heller, R. F. and Jacobs, H. S. (1978). Coronary heart disease in relation to age, sex, and the menopause. *Br. Med. J.*, **1**, 472

Johansson, B. W., Kaij, L., Kullander, S., Lenner, H. C., Svanberg, L. and Astedt, B. (1975). On some late effects of bilateral oophorectomy in the age range 15–30 years. *Acta Obstet. Gynecol. Scand.*, **54**, 449

P. A. van Keep, R. B. Greenblatt and M. Albeaux-Fernet (eds.) (1976). *Consensus on Menopause Research*. Proceedings of the First International Congress on the Menopause. (Lancaster: MTP Press)

P. A. van Keep and C. Lauritzen (eds.) (1973). *Ageing and Estrogens*. Front. Hormone Res., **2**. (Basel: Karger)

P. A. van Keep and C. Lauritzen (eds.) (1975). *Estrogens in the Post-menopause*. Front. Hormone Res., **3**. (Basel: Karger)

C. Lauritzen and P. A. van Keep (eds.) (1978). *Estrogen Therapy – The Benefits and Risks*. Front. Hormone Res., **5**. (Basel: Karger)

Lindsay, R., Aitken, J. M. and Anderson, J. B. (1976). Long-term prevention of post-menopausal osteoporosis by oestrogen. *Lancet*, **i**, 1038

Lindsay, R., Hart, D. M., Purdie, D., Ferguson, M. M., Clark, A. S. and Kraszewski, A. (1978). Comparative effects of oestrogen and a progestogen on bone loss in post-menopausal women. *Clin. Sci.*, **54**, 193

Recker, R. R., Saville, P. D. and Heaney, R. P. (1977). Effect of estrogens and calcium carbonate on bone loss in post-menopausal women. *Ann. Intern. Med.*, **87**, 649

Rosenberg, L., Armstrong, B. and Jick, H. (1976). Myocardial infarction and estrogen therapy in post-menopausal women. *N. Engl. J. Med.*, **294**, 1256

Thom, M., Chakravarti, S., Oram, D. and Studd, J. W. W. (1977). Effect of hormone replacement therapy on glucose tolerance in post-menopausal women. *Br. J. Obstet. Gynaecol.*, **84**, 776

Utian, W. H. (1968). Feminine forever? Current concepts of the menopause. A critical review. *S. Afr. J. Obstet. Gynaecol.*, **6**, 7

Utian, W. H. (1971). Cholesterol, coronary heart disease and oestrogens. *S. Afr. Med. J.*, **45**, 359

Utian, W. H. (1972). Effects of oophorectomy and oestrogen therapy on serum cholesterol. *Int. J. Gynecol. Obstet.*, **10**, 95

Utian, W. H. (1977). Current status of menopause and post-menopausal estrogen therapy. *Obstet. Gynecol. Surv.*, **32**, 193

Walters, S. and Jensen, H. K. (1977). Effect of treatment with oestradiol and oestriol on fasting serum cholesterol and triglyceride levels in post-menopausal women. *Br. J. Obstet. Gynaecol.*, **84**, 869

# Clotting factors and oestrogen replacement therapy

## Moderator: M. Notelovitz

Department of Obstetrics and Gynecology, University of Florida College of Medicine, Gainesville, Florida, USA

*Participants invited to present their views at this workshop included:*

*J. Bonnar (Ireland)*
*J. A. Davies (United Kingdom)*
*B.. Hochstädt (Israel)*
*H. Jick (USA)*
*E. S. Kohane (Israel)*
*J. W. W. Studd (United Kingdom)*
*M. I. Whitehead (United Kingdom)*

The workshop-session on clotting factors attempted three tasks: (a) an epidemiological assessment of the relationship between oestrogen replacement therapy in peri- and post-menopausal women and the development of certain thrombotic related vascular diseases, namely venous thrombosis, stroke and myocardial infarction, (b) a survey of current concepts of the mechanism of thrombosis and fibrinolysis as it relates to hormone replacement and finally, (c) the presentation of the most recent data on oestrogen replacement therapy and coagulation.

## EPIDEMIOLOGY

The epidemiological data presented (Jick) were based on the Boston Collaborative Drug Surveillance Program which had collected information from over 60 000 hospitalized medical and surgical patients. Included was information on menopausal status, drug intake, personal habits and discharge diagnosis. The data were organized and analysed in order to evaluate the relationship of exogenous oestrogen therapy, patient characteristics, and the menopause itself, to various vascular illnesses.

To set the epidemiological picture in perspective, data was first presented relating to the association between oral contraceptive use and 'idiopathic' thrombosis. Thus, compared with non-users, the estimate of relative risk for thromboembolism in oral contraceptive users is 11, and the estimated attack-rate attributable to oral contraceptives is 60 per 100 000 users per year. The relative risk estimate for stroke among oral contraceptive users compared with non-users is 26. Cigarette smoking is only weakly associated with stroke in this group of women. The relative risk estimate for the development of myocardial infarction comparing oral contraceptive users with non-users is 14. In this category, all but two patients (out of a total of 26 subjects) were cigarette smokers. While this illness is rare in most healthy young women, the risk in women older than about 37 years who both smoke and take oral contraceptives appears to be high (Jick et al., 1978).

The possible influence of oestrogen-containing drugs (mainly conjugated oestrogens) on venous thromboembolism in post-menopausal women 45–69 years of age was explored. Significant associations between oestrogens and idiopathic venous thromboembolism were not present. Data were also examined to determine the risk of non-fatal acute myocardial infarction in post-menopausal women 40–75 years of age in relation to the use of oestrogen-containing drugs. Once again no statistically significant association could be found (Rosenberg et al., 1976).

Two further pertinent points arose from this epidemiological survey: (a) there does not appear to be an association between an operative menopause, or premature menopause, and the risk of hospitalization for acute myocardial infarction, and (b) cigarette smoking is positively correlated with an earlier onset of the menopause (Jick et al., 1977). In evaluating women aged 44–47 years, the age-standardized proportions of women who were post-menopausal were 35, 36, 43 and 49% respectively for never smokers, ex-smokers, and current smokers of half to one pack, or more per day.

## HORMONES AND COAGULATION

The changes that occur in the initiation and dissolution of clot formation were outlined, and the role of platelets, and the various factors of the coagulation cascade and the all-important fibrinolytic system were discussed. With regard to the latter, two factors were emphasized both of which may be adversely affected by oestrogen replacement therapy, namely, anti-thrombin III, a naturally occurring anti-coagulant said to be responsible for 75% of the natural fluidity of blood, and the fibrinolytic system in the vascular endothelium.

In surveying the vast literature on the effect of oral contraceptives on coagulation, it was noted that, whilst some factors, VII and X for example, do indeed appear to increase, the increase is small when compared with the changes that are found during pregnancy, and that pregnancy is not really associated with a significant risk of serious thrombotic episodes.

Further emphasis was made regarding the fact that laboratory observed increases or decreases in the coagulation profile, does not infer that the patient will be liable to thrombotic or bleeding tendencies.

With regard to the effects of oestrogen replacement therapy in peri-menopausal women, it was noted that, despite the increase in clotting factors associated with ageing, natural oestrogens – oestradiol valerate and conjugated oestrogens – induce relatively little change in most of the coagulation factors studied. The same was not true for the use of synthetic oestrogen – mestranol – and it was suggested that the use of this preparation may provide a thrombogenic hazard.

A cautious note was struck, and it was suggested that before a definitive conclusion could be reached, long-term prospective clinical studies should be undertaken, which, together with the expansion of present epidemiological surveys, should mean the avoidance of the experience gained with oral contraceptives and their association with inappropriate thrombosis (Notelovitz, 1977).

105

## CLINICAL TRIALS

Four investigators presented findings from clinical trials. Experience with the use of a variety of different oestrogens and combination therapies was summarized (Studd). Patients were divided into six groups and given conjugated equine oestrogen (Premarin), oestradiol valerate (Progynova), piperazine oestrone sulphate (Harmogen), Serial 28 – a sequential ethinyl oestradiol with megestrol acetate, ethynodiol diacetate or an oestradiol/testosterone implant with cyclical norethisterone. The results showed: (1) a change in kaolin-cephalin clotting time only with ethynodiol acetate, (2) no significant change in the platelet count in any group, (3) an increase in fibrino-lytic activity as demonstrated by the development of fibrin degra-dation products in nine of the 33 patients, (4) no significant changes in platelet aggregation in patients on Premarin, Progynova or implants, and (5) an increase in platelet aggregation after Harmogen and Serial 28 therapy, and a decrease after ethynodiol diacetate therapy. Thus, once again, none of the so-called natural oestrogens produced significantly changed parameters in the clotting profile. Further, the route of administration may also be important, as patients treated with implants did not have a significant change in any of the coagulation parameters studied despite assumed adequate/high oestrogen levels (Thom et al., 1978).

The role of long-term therapy and its effect on coagulation was reported (Davies). The preparation used was oestriol succinate and patients were studied for 12 months. The only notable changes were increased concentrations of euglobulin lysis activity, increasing plasma concentrations of plasminogen, and an increase in platelet aggregation to collagen. It could be concluded that, despite epidemiological evidence relating oestrogen administration and thrombotic disease, oestriol succinate was less likely to have an adverse effect on blood coagulation than synthetic oestrogens given in an apparently equivalent dosage (Toy et al., 1978).

The third study reported was one relating to the recovery of clotting factors subsequent to oestrogen medication (Kohane and Hochstädt). The blood clotting systems of 542 female patients were investigated by repeated determinations of fibrinogen, prothrombin time, factors V and VII, and anti-thrombin III activity. All were performed prior to, during and subsequent to oestrogen treatment. It was concluded that anti-thrombin III activity was the most reliable and sensitive test – with this test both the earliest alterations and restoration of the clotting system was revealed. A significant drop in anti-thrombin III appeared as early as the 7th day of oestrogen therapy. The length of the recovery period of anti-thrombin III activity from cessation of oestrogen replacement therapy varied significantly depending on the type of oestrogen employed. It lasted 14–21 days in women who had received synthetic oestrogen preparations and only 7–12 days in those treated with conjugated oestrogens.

The relationship between leg cramps, oestrogen replacement therapy and deep venous thrombosis, was the subject of a double-blind cross-over study with conjugated oestrogen 1.25 mg, administered cyclically, and alternating with a placebo, each for periods of 3 months (Whitehead). The radioactive-labelled fibrinogen test was used to screen the patients for inappropriate venous thrombosis. The principal finding of this study was that although there was a significant increase in leg cramps when the patients were on oestrogen replacement therapy – this was reported by 20% of the test group – no instances of venous thrombosis were detected.

## DISCUSSION

Discussion of the above papers covered a wide range of aspects of oestrogen replacement therapy and thrombosis. One of the questions posed was whether a laboratory test existed which could predict or monitor the asymptomatic development of a hyper-coagulable state. Some of the participants felt that anti-thrombin III or anti-Xa could be used for this purpose. Studd had used an automated, but sensitive, anti-Xa assay to measure changes before and during oestrogen replacement therapy. To date all 600 patients have shown anti-Xa activity within normal levels. However, even with the acknowledged present deficiencies, monitoring of anti-thrombin III activity is still the most promising and practical test available. It appeared from the presented data, that the apparent lack of adverse effect of oestrogen replacement therapy compared with the use of oestrogen-containing oral contraceptives, related to the type of oestrogens used. In addition, it was suggested that the route of administration may be of importance in that avoidance of the entero-hepatic circulation may in some way confer a lesser liability of exogenous oestrogens to induce a hyper-coagulable state. This area needs further research.

The 'biological potency' of the oestrogen used may also be a reason for these disparate results (between oestrogen replacement therapy and oral contraceptives). Unfortunately there are no satisfactory means of assessing this point at present; a study is currently being conducted at the University of Florida in which the levels of oestrone, oestradiol, oestriol, sex-binding globulin and the pituitary gonadotropins are being measured in relation to the clotting profile of menopausal women on different types and doses of oestrogen replacement therapy.

Apart from their effect on clotting, oestrogens may indeed have significant effects on blood flow and.on the integrity of the vascular endothelium. In this way, oestrogen replacement therapy may contribute to the pathogenesis of thrombus formation. More research is also needed in this area.

Whereas doubts existed regarding the precise role of oestrogens in the induction of clot formation, it was generally agreed that smoking had a direct cause and effect relationship to, e.g. the development of myocardial infarction. Patients on oestrogen replacement therapy should therefore be actively discouraged from smoking.

The possibility of a protective effect of progestogens if given simultaneously with oestrogen replacement therapy was put forward. There is, however, no work to confirm this concept at present.

## IN CONCLUSION

To summarize the proceedings of the session on clotting factors, it may be said that until further epidemiological evidence is presented hormone replacement therapy, using natural oestrogens in healthy menopausal women who do not smoke, is unlikely to result in a significant increase in inappropriate thrombosis and the resulting vascular diseases of myocardial infarction, stroke and deep vein thrombosis.

## References

Jick, H., Porter, J. and Morrison, A. S. (1977). Relation between smoking and age of natural menopause. *Lancet*, **i**, 1354

Jick, H., Dinan, B. and Rothman, K. J. (1978). Oral contraceptives and non-fatal myocardial infarctions. *J. Am. Med. Assoc.*, **239**, 1403

Notelovitz, M. (1977). Coagulation, oestrogen, and the menopause. In: *Clinics in Obstetrics and Gynaecology* (R. B. Greenblatt and J. W. W. Studd, eds.), vol. 4, p. 107. (London: Saunders)

Rosenberg, L., Armstrong, B. and Jick, H. (1976). Myocardial infarction and oestrogen therapy in post-menopausal women. *N. Engl. J. Med.,* **294**, 1256

Thom, M., Dubiel, M., Kakkar, V. V. and Studd, J. W. W. (1978). The effect of different regimens of oestrogens on the clotting and fibrinolytic system of post-menopausal women. In: *Estrogen Therapy – The Benefits and Risks. Front. Hormone Res.* (C. Lauritzen and P. A. van Keep, eds.), **5**, 192

Toy, J. L., Davies, J. A. and McNicol, G. P. (1978). The effect of long-term therapy with oestriol succinate on the haemostatic mechanism in post-menopausal women. *Br. J. Obstet. Gynaecol.,* **88**, 363

# The endometrium in the menopause

## Moderator: S. Campbell

## Secretary: M. I. Whitehead

Department of Obstetrics and Gynaecology, King's College Hospital
Medical School, London, United Kingdom

*Participants invited to present their views at this
workshop included:*

*D. W. Cramer (USA)*
*R. D. Gambrell, Jr (USA)*
*R. J. B. King (United Kingdom)*
*M. E. L. Paterson (United Kingdom)*
*D. R. Shanklin (USA)*
*M. I. Whitehead (United Kingdom)*

## INTRODUCTION

The effects of exogenous oestrogens on the endometrium have
become of special significance to both the medical and lay public.
Oestrogens have been suggested as an aetiological factor in the
development of endometrial cancer, thus causing concern to
physicians; and sensational handling by the media of any reported
oestrogen/cancer link, however ill- or well-founded, inevitably
distresses patients. Few topics provoke more discussion amongst
well-informed clinicians and the resultant controversy only confuses
the non-expert medical practitioner.

The aims of the histologist, epidemiologist, biochemist and three clinicians who participated in this session were to define the sources of error in interpretation of endometrial histology, to review the epidemiological evidence suggesting an oestrogen/cancer relationship, and to present histological and biochemical evidence indicating that the potential hazards of oestrogens can be reduced.

## ENDOMETRIAL HISTOLOGY

### Errors in sample collection and histological reporting

All clinical interpretation of endometrial tissue obtained at curettage should allow for two possible sources of error – those of sampling, and inconsistencies in histological reporting.

Errors in sampling usually result in under-diagnosis of malign lesions. They arise because the pathological areas are not included in the biopsy specimen. For example, curettage, especially outpatient suction curettage which is widely used in clinical studies, may fail to remove basal endometrium and this may be the only area showing dysplastic change. Furthermore, many pathological lesions, whether hyperplastic or malignant, are focal and may be missed because curettage removes at most only 50% of endometrial tissue. This is especially important during oestrogen therapy which may cause the development of all degrees of hyperplasia. The variation in histology may be such that it is possible to obtain relatively normal proliferative endometrium from one area of the uterine cavity, and severe atypical hyperplasia from another.

Errors in histological reporting invariably result in over-diagnosis of hyperplasia for carcinoma. They arise because during oestrogen therapy morphological variation is great and interpretation is to some extent subjective. When uncertainty exists error is biased towards clinical caution, malignancy is over-recorded (Greenblatt et al., 1966), and surgery undertaken. The differentiation between severe atypical hyperplasia and adenocarcinoma may be very difficult histologically as both can exhibit mitotic figures, infolding of epithelium and 'back to back' gland formation. The true distinction may have to be made functionally with administration of progestogens and repeat curettage. Severe atypia will reverse to secretory endometrium, carcinoma will not (Greenblatt, 1976).

Inappropriate histological evaluation undoubtedly occurred in some of the retrospective studies reporting an increase of cancer following prolonged oestrogen therapy and was a serious methodological weakness. Subsequent review has indicated an incidence of over-diagnosis of approximately 20% in some studies and the same figure has been quoted by Szekely *et al*. (1978). However, the latter authors concluded that over-recording of malignancy can account for only a small part of the rising incidence of endometrial carcinoma.

## Endometrial hyperplasia

The relationship between spontaneously arising hyperplasia and endometrial carcinoma is well-founded upon extensive documentation and the literature has been reviewed (Gusberg, 1976). Estimates of the risks of the subsequent development of cancer range from 1% with cystic glandular hyperplasia (McBride, 1959) to 45% with severe atypia (Campbell and Barter, 1961); and the best designed study reported a cumulative risk of 30% at 10 years over controls (Gusberg and Kaplan, 1963).

Preliminary data from a descriptive study of the age distribution of the various types of hyperplasia and cancer suggest that the progression from hyperplasia to malignancy usually takes between 10 and 20 years, and that focal hyperplasia can arise as early as 35 years of age (Shanklin, 1976).

## REVIEW OF THE EPIDEMIOLOGICAL EVIDENCE

Epidemiological studies on oestrogens and endometrial carcinoma may be divided into two broad categories – descriptive and aetiological.

*Descriptive studies* have provided evidence for a relationship but should not be interpreted as showing causality. For example, Greenwald *et al*. (1977) related the increase in oestrogen sales in up-state New York in the late 1960s and early 1970s to the observed increase in the incidence of carcinoma. It has been pointed out, however, that there has, as yet, been no increase in mortality in these areas but for reasons that are discussed below no such rise may be seen.

*Aetiological studies* are necessary to define causes or at least risk factors for disease. The five published case-control studies (Smith *et al*., 1975; Ziel and Finkle, 1975; Mack *et al*., 1976; Gray *et al*.,

1977; McDonald *et al.*, 1977) all reported an increase in risk for endometrial carcinoma with oestrogen use of 6 or more months. The best estimate for this risk from these studies is 5.0 (95% confident limits: 4.0–6.2). Because of methodological biases and inadequacies the studies have been criticized and comprehensive repetition is beyond the scope of this report. Much that was most incisive in this forum appeared in invited editorials and reviews (Gordan and Greenberg, 1976; Kistner, 1976; Feinstein and Horwitz, 1977; Mack and Pike, 1977; Berger and Fowler, 1977; Barron, 1978).

In summary, the criticisms were concentrated on observation bias, selection bias, confounding factors, and misinterpretation of histology. The latter has been considered previously.

Observation bias results in mis-classification of either non-exposed invididuals as exposed or vice versa; or non-diseased individuals as diseased and vice versa. It is feasible that details of previous oestrogen use in cancer-sufferers were obtained more carefully than those of the controls. However, this type of bias is unlikely to have distorted the results of three of the studies where histories were collected from medication records made prior to diagnosis.

Selection bias infers that cases have in some way been selected on a correlate of exposure. It has been proposed that diseased women who have taken oestrogens *co-incidentally* are more likely to be diagnosed than cancer sufferers not so exposed. However, for selection bias to have accounted for the strong dose and duration-dependent oestrogen/cancer link reported it must be shown that: first there is a large pool of undiagnosed cancer in the community and second that accessibility to diagnostic procedure is increased with dose and duration of drug usage. Both are improbable. Selection bias is likely to be minimal when accessibility to medical care is similar for both cases and controls – as in the retirement community of Mack *et al.* (1976) and the private practice of Gray *et al.* (1977).

A confounding factor is associated with both the disease and exposure. For example, higher socio-economic status is associated with increased risk of carcinoma perhaps due to obesity; in the United States it is also associated with better health care and therefore increased use of oestrogens for menopausal symptoms. Confounding bias can be reduced by selecting homogenous populations for study, by matching cases and controls for confounding factors, and by stratifying during analysis. All five studies used one or more of these techniques. Furthermore, although the control groups were divergent, the reported increased risk between studies was fairly consistent and this suggests that inadequate control selection cannot entirely account for the findings.

Bias from mis-classification, selection, and confounding therefore may have falsely elevated the reported risk but it is unlikely to have produced a spurious result. Furthermore, a direct drug effect is suggested by increasing risk with greater dosage or oestrogen and by increased duration of usage. Whilst conjugated oestrogen was the most commonly prescribed preparation, increased risk was also reported with intra-muscular and other oral oestrogens, including non-steroidal therapy.

At present it is unclear whether the association between increase in risk and duration of usage is linear or exponential as both types of regression curve can be fitted equally well to the available evidence. The implications, however, are quite different. In a linear relationship the increase in risk rises by a factor of approximately one per annum; in the exponential model the risk remains relatively small for the first 3–4 years of oestrogen usage, but thereafter doubles every 3 years.

Finally, and very importantly, oestrogen use appeared to be more strongly linked to the early, less invasive cancers (Stage I) and weakest for the more invasive (Stages II–IV). The implication is that the aetiology of the more advanced lesions may be largely unaccounted for by drug use. As the more superficial cancers are those with the most favourable prognosis and greater survival, an increase in the incidence of cancer is most unlikely to result in a similar rise in mortality. It is for this reason that the benefits of therapy may well out-weigh the potential hazards from carcinoma.

## CLINICAL STUDIES

Gambrell reported 2 years' prospective and 1 year's retrospective work. The majority of patients took orally either unopposed oestrogens, oestrogen with progestogen, or were untreated. A smaller group received either androgens, progestogens or oestrogens topically. Thirteen adenocarcinomas were diagnosed in a total of 8170 years of patient observation, giving an overall incidence rate of 1.6 : 1000 post-menopausal women per year.

The highest incidence rate, 3.8 per 1000 women-years was found in the group receiving unopposed oestrogens orally (8 cancers per 2088 years of observation) and the lowest, 0.3 per 1000 women-years, in women receiving oral oestrogen/progestogen therapy (1 cancer per 3792 years of observation). This difference was statistically significant ($p < 0.01$). In untreated women the incidence rate was 2.0 per 1000 women-years and one adenocarcinoma was detected in 775 years of observation in the smaller group receiving other hormones (incidence rate 1.3 per 1000 women-years). This one patient had been using topical oestrogens.

Of the well-recognized predisposing factors for endometrial carcinoma, only two – low parity and endometrial hyperplasia – were to be found in six or more of the 13 cancer patients. Eight patients were Para 1 or less; cystic hyperplasia was found in three patients, and atypical hyperplasia in a further three patients from 4 months to 8 years prior to the development of cancer. The one patient to develop carcinoma during oestrogen/progestogen therapy was one of the three initially diagnosed as having atypical hyperplasia; progestogens had been prescribed for 5 days each calendar month.

Gambrell also reported reversal of hyperplasia to normal endometrium in 192 out of 199 patients (96.8%) following progestogen course. The results suggested that C19 progestogens might be more efficient in this respect than C21 progestogens.

The protective effect of progestogens was further emphasized by Whitehead and Paterson both of whom presented histological data obtained by serial endometrial biopsy from prospective longitudinal on-going trials. Whitehead reported that after a mean duration of 16 months, the incidence of hyperplasia with cyclical unopposed oestrogens was 32% at high-dose (the maximum manufacturers' recommended dosage) and 16% at low dose. Addition of a progestogen for 5 or 7 days each calendar month reduced this incidence to 4% with high-dose regimens and 3% with low-dose regimens and this reduction was significant ($p < 0.001$). Two-thirds of these cases were cystic hyperplasia and the remainder atypical hyperplasia.

In Paterson's study, of shorter duration, the equivalent figure for combined high and low dosage unopposed oestrogen was 14%, one-sixth of which was adenomatous or atypical. The overall incidence of hyperplasia during oral sequential therapy was 2% but importantly, no case of hyperplasia arose in 133 patients given

116

progestogens for 10 or more days each month. Greater numbers are required to determine whether 10-day regimens are totally effective in protecting against the development of hyperplasia. During implant therapy progestogens were added for 5 days each month and the least satisfactory results were obtained – the incidence of hyperplasia being 22%. This is perhaps attributable to problems with patient compliance as progestin ingestion may cause unpleasant side-effects, such as headache, backache, abdominal discomfort or vaginal bleeding. Such problems deserve urgent consideration as there is little point prescribing a progestin that has a suppressant effect on hyperplasia but which causes adverse symptoms and disturbs other biological parameters.

Both trials showed that during unopposed cyclical oestrogen therapy, vaginal bleeding was wholly unreliable as an indicator of endometrial pathology. Normal endometrium and hyperplasia were both found in association with scheduled withdrawal bleeding, unscheduled break-through bleeding, and no vaginal bleeding. With oestrogen/progestogen regimens, regular withdrawal bleeding invariably occurred with a normal endometrium but did not absolutely exclude pathology; break-through bleeding was more likely to be associated with pathology and therefore required immediate investigation.

These results strongly indicate that serial biopsies are required on all patients receiving either oestrogen or oestrogen/progestogen regimens. Curettage should be repeated during cyclical therapy at yearly intervals at the very minimum; and as on present evidence the protection afforded by progestogen is incomplete, curettage should be performed at intervals of 12 to 18 months during sequential treatment.

Whitehead again emphasized that hyperplasia may pre-date therapy but may be unsuspected as abnormal vaginal bleeding may not have occurred. Both patients who developed carcinoma in his study had pre-existing hyperplasia. He also considered 'hormone replacement therapy' an inappropriate term as all oral exogenous oestrogens, whether oestrone or oestradiol preparations, did not rectify the post-menopausal plasma deficiency of oestradiol but gave rise principally to oestrone, and resulted in urinary total oestrogen excretion in and above the pre-menopausal mid-cycle ovulatory range. The development of hyperplasia was thought to be totally explained by these findings.

117

Preliminary reports from these clinical studies have been published (Gambrell, 1977a, 1977b, and 1978; Whitehead *et al.*, 1977; Whitehead and Campbell, 1978; Whitehead, 1978; Sturdee *et al.*, 1978).

## BIOCHEMICAL STUDIES

Despite being repeatedly advocated, prospective randomized controlled clinical trials to determine the exact risk of cancer with oestrogen therapy have still not commenced. In the United Kingdom the Medical Research Council have decided that such trials would be impracticable in view of the relatively small number of women receiving such treatment. If such a trial was started now many years would elapse before reliable data emerged. Therefore, other approaches to rapidly determine the regimens affording greatest endometrial protection must be sought. One such approach is the study of cell biochemistry.

King investigated endometrial tissue obtained in the Whitehead trial and reported on changes in nuclear oestrogen and cytoplasmic progesterone receptor levels, qualitative intranuclear oestrogen concentrations, and oestradiol-17$\beta$ dehydrogenase activity.

During cyclical unopposed oestrogen and sequential oestrogen/progestogen regimens nuclear oestrogen and cytoplasmic progesterone receptor levels were within the pre-menopausal proliferative phase range for 2 of every 4-week treatment schedules. Therefore, the oestrogenic stimulus being applied to the endometrium is potent.

The inclusion of the progestogen, norethisterone, affected the receptor machinery in three ways. First, the amount of nuclear oestrogen receptor was lowered. Second, the proportion of total cellular oestrogen receptor was reduced, and third the proportion of oestradiol relative to oestrone in the nucleus was lowered. These three effects probably result in part from norethisterone inducing oestradiol-17$\beta$ dehydrogenase. This enzyme primarily converts oestradiol to oestrone, thus decreasing the effective affinity of intracellular oestrogen for the receptor and lowering its biological effectiveness. Although during exogenous oestrogen therapy the plasma oestrone to oestradiol ratio ranges from 2–5 : 1 in favour of oestrone, direct analysis of nuclear oestrogen concentrations showed an excess of oestradiol to oestrone by 5–6 : 1. During the period of progestin administration, this was reduced to 2–3 : 1. This indicates that in the post-menopausal woman receiving oestrogens, oestradiol is the active intracellular oestrogen.

Preliminary reports of this work have been published (King *et al.*, 1978a and 1978b).

## CONCLUSIONS

Sampling and reporting errors must always be taken into account when endometrial histology is being interpreted.

The epidemiological evidence suggests a true link between un-opposed exogenous oestrogens and the early less-invasive forms of endometrial adeno-carcinoma.

Hyperplasia, a pre-malignant condition, results from unopposed oestrogen therapy and its development cannot be predicted from the bleeding pattern.

Progestogens appear capable of protecting against the development of cancer and hyperplasia, although complete protection has still to be achieved.

At cellular level, progestins interfere with receptor machinery, the means whereby oestrogens stimulate the cell.

## References

Barron, B. A. (1978). Exogenous estrogen and endometrial cancer: a statistical problem. *Contemporary Obstet. Gynecol.*, **11**, 135

Berger, G. S. and Fowler, W. C. (1977). Exogenous oestrogens and endometrial carcinoma: a review and comments for the clinician. *J. Reprod. Med.*, **18**, 177

Campbell, P. E. and Barter, G. A. (1961). The significance of atypical hyperplasia. *J. Obstet. Gynaecol. Br. Cwlth.*, **68**, 668

Feinstein, A. R. and Horwitz, R. I. (1977). An analytic critique of five studies investigating the relationship of estrogens and endometrial cancer. Presented to the *American Society for Clinical Investigation*, 1 May, Washington, DC, USA

Gambrell, R. D. Jr. (1977a). Estrogens, progestogens and endometrial cancer. *J. Reprod. Med.*, **18**, 6, 301

Gambrell, R. D. Jr. (1977b). Postmenopausal bleeding. In: *Clinics in Obstetrics and Gynaecology* (R. B. Greenblatt and J. W. W. Studd, eds.), **4**, 1, 129. (London: Saunders)

Gambrell, R. D. Jr. (1978). The prevention of endometrial cancer in post-menopausal women with progestogens. *Maturitas*, **1**, 107

Gordan, G. S. and Greenberg, B. G. (1976). Exogenous estrogens and endometrial cancer. *Postgrad Med.*, **59**, 66

Gray; L. A. Snr., Christopherson, W. M. and Hoover, R. N. (1977). Estrogens and endometrial carcinoma. *Obstet. Gynecol.*, **49**, 385

Greenblatt, R. B. (1976). Estrogens and endometrial cancer. In: *The Menopause* (R. J. Beard, ed.), p. 247. (Lancaster: MTP Press)

Greenblatt, R. B., Stoddard, L. and King, P. (1966). Estrogen in endometrial carcinogenesis. In: *New Concepts in Gynecological Oncology* (G. C.·Lewis, Jr, W. B. Wentz and R. M. Jaffe, eds.). (Philadelphia: F. A. Davis)

Greenwald, P., Caputo, T. A. and Wolfgand, P. E. (1977). Endometrial cancer after menopausal use of estrogens. *Obstet. Gynecol.*, **50**, 239

Gusberg, S. B. (1976). The individual at high risk for endometrial carcinoma. *Am. J. Obstet. Gynecol.*, **126**, 535

Gusberg, S. B. and Kaplan, A. (1963). Precursors of corpus carcinoma IV. Adenomatous hyperplasia as Stage 0 carcinoma of the endometrium. *Am. J. Obstet. Gynecol.*, **87**, 662

King, R. J. B., Whitehead, M. I., Campbell, S. and Minardi, J. (1978a). Biochemical studies on endometrium from post-menopausal women receiving hormone replacement therapy. *Postgrad. Med. J.*, **54**, (Suppl. 2), 65

King, R. J. B., Whitehead, M. I., Campbell, S. and Minardi, J. (1978b). Effects of oestrogens and progestin on the biochemistry of the post-menopausal endometrium. In: *The Role of Oestrogen/Progestogen Therapy in the Management of the Menopause* (I. D. Cooke, ed.). (Lancaster: MTP Press)

Kistner, R. W. (1976). Estrogens and endometrial cancer. *Obstet. Gynecol.*, **48**, 479

Mack, T. M. and Pike, M. C. (1977). Hormone replacement therapy and endometrial carcinoma. *Lancet*, **ii**, 1358

Mack, T., Pike, M., Henderson, B., Pfeffer, R., Gerkins, V., Arthur, M. and Brown, S. (1976). Estrogens and endometrial cancer in a retirement community. *N. Engl. J. Med.*, **294**, 1262

McBride, J. M. (1959). Pre-menopausal cystic hyperplasia and endometrial carcinoma. *J. Obstet. Gynaecol. Br. Emp.*, **66**, 288

McDonald, T. W., Annegers, J. F., O'Fallan, W. M., Dockerty, M. B., Malkasian, G. D. and Kurland, L. T. (1977). Exogenous estrogen and endometrial carcinoma: Case control and incidence study. *Am. J. Obstet. Gynecol.*, **127**, 572

Shanklin, D. R. (1976). Estrogens and endometrial carcinoma. *N. Engl. J. Med.*, **294**, 847

Smith, D. C., Prentice, R., Thompson, D. and Herrman, W. (1975). Association of exogenous oestrogens and endometrial carcinoma. *N. Engl. J. Med.*, **293**, 1164

Sturdee, D. W., Wade-Evans, T., Paterson, M. E. L., Thom, M. and Studd, J. W. W. (1978). Relations between bleeding pattern, endometrial histology and oestrogen treatment in menopausal women. *Br. Med. J.*, **1**, 1575

Szekely, D. R., Weiss, M. S. and Schweld, A. I. (1978). Incidence of endometrial carcinoma in King County, Washington: a standardized histological review. *J. Nat. Cancer Inst.*, **60**, 985

Whitehead, M. I. (1978). The effects of oestrogens and progestogens on the post-menopausal endometrium. *Maturitas*, **1**, 87

Whitehead, M. I. and Campbell, S. (1978). Endometrial histology, uterine bleeding and oestrogen levels in menopausal women receiving oestrogen therapy and oestrogen/progestogen therapy. In: *Proceedings of the Second International Meeting on Endometrial Cancer and Allied Topics* (M. J. Brush, R. W. Taylor, R. J. King, eds.). (London: Ballière Tindall)

Whitehead, M. I., McQueen, J., Beard, R. J., Minardi, J. and Campbell, S. (1977). The effects of cyclical oestrogen therapy and sequential oestrogen/progestogen therapy on the endometrium of post-menopausal women. *Acta Obstet. Gynecol. Scand.* (Suppl. 65), 91

Ziel, H. and Finkle, W. (1975). Increased risk of endometrial carcinoma among users of conjugated estrogens. *N. Engl. J. Med.*, **293**, 1167

# Management of the patient, including the high-risk patient

## Moderator: C. Lauritzen

Department of Gynaecology and Obstetrics, University of Ulm,
West Germany

*Participants invited to present their views at this
workshop included:*

*R. B. Greenblatt (USA)*
*A. A. Haspels (The Netherlands)*
*H. M. Lemon (USA)*
*D. McKay Hart (United Kingdom)*
*D. M. Serr (Israel)*
*J. W. W. Studd (United Kingdom)*
*W. H. Utian (USA)*

Successful treatment depends on the right medicament being
prescribed for a specific disorder. When treating climacteric and
post-climacteric complaints, the prescribing physician will be guided
by the symptoms presented and by the character of the patient – the
type of woman she is – when he is selecting the drug, the dose, the
mode of administration, and the frequency of administration. Thereafter, the medication should be continued as long as is necessary,
but no longer than is sensible.

All highly effective medicaments, and oestrogens and progestogens come into this category, also exert strong side-effects. The side-
effects which may occur should be anticipated, and then prevented

121

or minimized as much as possible in order that the patients may enjoy the benefits of the therapy without suffering, or being inconvenienced by, the adverse side-effects.

## INDIVIDUALIZATION OF TREATMENT

The variety of different hormone preparations available, either as single substances or in combinations, means that it is possible for therapies to be specially devised for individual patients. In making his selection, the physician will take into account the personal history of the patient, the results of the physical examination, the pattern of complaints, the indications for treatment, the contraindications and risk factors, the aim of the therapy, and last but not least the wishes of the patient herself. Acceptability of the therapy by the patient depends on the good effects of the therapy on her symptoms and complaints, on the absence or insignificance of side-effects, and on the convenience of the treatment. When a patient regards a therapy as satisfactory in these respects, her co-operation and motivation to continue with the treatment will be assured.

## SIDE-EFFECTS

Subjective side-effects are to be separated from objective ones. From the physician's viewpoint, the most frequently occurring subjective side-effects of oestrogen therapy are breast discomfort and a feeling of tension in the legs. Breast discomfort, incidentally, is often an early indication of an over-dosage of oestrogen. Objective side-effects are oedema, uterine bleedings, and, in a few cases, weight gain. In some cases the oral administration *per se* of the oestrogen medication causes nausea and gastrointestinal complaints such as bloating. Many side-effects, such as hypertension, hypertriglycerid-aemia, changes in clotting factor levels, and hyperproliferation of the endometrium, can, of course, only be detected by special diagnostic measures.

The side-effect which causes the greatest number of drop outs from therapy is post-menopausal uterine bleeding. In recent years some women have also stopped therapy because of fears of thrombosis and cancer – fears which are often the result of reports in newspapers or of gossip, but which are sometimes induced by doctors.

## DETERMINANTS OF SIDE-EFFECTS

The effects and side-effects of oestrogen therapy are dose-dependent. High dosages and overdosages are among the main causes of undesired side-effects. Others are acyclic medication (which can lead to cumulation), the duration of the treatment, an unsuitable mode of administration, the addition of other hormones, the presence of risk factors, and the patient's psychology.

A dose-dependent relationship has been shown for hyperproliferation of the endometrium with atypical uterine bleedings, painful breasts, oedema, rapid weight gain, coagulation changes, some plasma lipid changes, an increase of bromsulphalein retention, and alterations in glucose metabolism. The existence of this dose–response relationship is also evidenced by the fact that an increase in dosage usually raises the incidence of these side-effects, whereas a simple decrease often results in their reduction or even disappearance. A clear example of this is seen regarding vascular complications in women taking oestrogens in oral contraceptives or for the postpartum inhibition of lactation, and in men taking oestrogens after a myocardial infarction and for prostatic cancer.

The oral administration *per se* of oestrogens can also cause adverse side-effects as when oestrogens are administered in this way they can cause local gastrointestinal problems, and, because of their early passage through the liver, strongly and unnecessarily stimulate biosynthetic activity in this organ.

Other side-effects are induced by the use of artificial oestrogens, such as mestranol and ethinyl oestradiol. These are a burden for liver metabolism, can cause cholestasis because of C-17 alkylation, and, because of a strong and prolonged half-life and reduced clearance, may cumulate if given daily for a long period of time.

It is now fairly clear, however, that the most important cause of the undesired side-effects of oestrogen therapy is the inability of the treatment as it is used at the present time to imitate completely normal glandular oestrogen-progesterone secretion. This is particularly true when the oestrogens are administered orally, for then, because of the variations in resorption and of the intestinal metabolism prior to uptake, the plasma levels are atypical. Accordingly, other means of therapeutic administration are again under consideration; these include intramuscular injections, the implantation of pellets, and percutaneous, buccal, vaginal and rectal applications.

123

There are many points to be resolved before firm recommendations can be made in this respect. It has already been shown, however, that percutaneous administration can lead to oestrogen levels which are comparable to those seen during the normal cycle, and that vaginal administration results in a high proportion. With both methods the blood plasma levels appear to be more physiological than after oral ingestion, with the oestradiol concentration being higher than that of oestrone.

## ADDITION OF A PROGESTOGEN OR OF AN ANDROGEN

The synergistic actions of certain progestogens and androgens make it possible to reduce the amount of oestrogens used for the treatment of climacteric complaints. Androgens, for instance, can enhance the psychotropic effects of oestrogens, a factor which can make their administration useful in cases of depression (Greenblatt). Androgens and nortestosterone-progestogens act synergistically with oestrogens in correcting urinary stress incontinence. Some androgens, as well as norethisterone and norgestrel, can counter a triglyceride increasing activity of oestrogens. Other effects are inhibition of cervical hyper-secretion, relief from breast tension and mastopathia, and the prevention of the growth of myoma, and of endometriosis; they also inhibit hyperproliferation due to oestrogens, induce secretory trans-formation, and, upon withdrawal, prompt the shedding of the endometrium. Thus, in certain cases, the administration of a pro-gestogen or of an androgen along with the oestrogen is advisable.

Progestogens and androgens can, however, also exert undesired effects. Progestogens may inhibit the positive psychotropic effects of oestrogens and lead to a feeling of tiredness and even of depression. They sometimes decrease libido, cause oedema, weight increase, and slight hirsutism. Androgens also sometimes induce hirsutism, and can cause acne, seborrhoea, a deepening of the voice, hyper-trophy of the clitoris, and, sometimes, an undesired increase in libido.

## INDICATIONS FOR AN ANDROGEN–OESTROGEN TREATMENT OF CLIMACTERIC COMPLAINTS

A depressive mood which does not respond well to oestrogens alone, a loss of drive and activity, psychasthenia, anorgasmia, loss of weight

124

and of libido are all conditions which can often be improved by the administration of an androgen–oestrogen combination therapy. The use of the adrenal steroid dehydroepiandrosterone (prasterone) may also be considered. This is a very weak androgen, which exerts an anticatabolic and slight psychotropic effect.

## DOSE DISTRIBUTION

Memory packages have been developed in an attempt to ensure the intake of the exact replacement dose every day. There is, however, also a place for an individualized therapy. For instance, a high dose in the first days of the treatment cycle followed by a low protracted dose will prevent an unwanted endometrial bleeding, and a 'never at weekends' dosage scheme may reduce side-effects caused by cumulation. Satisfactory results have also been achieved with the so-called 'lazy medication' system whereby the patient takes a tablet according to her own judgement of when one is needed.

## DURATION OF TREATMENT

The treatment should be given as long as is necessary, but no longer than is sensible. This means that therapy should be given as long as it is relieving climacteric complaints, and as long as the prophylactic effects on osteoporosis and on the urogenital targets and skin are desired, but that it should be discontinued if contra-indications arise and in extreme old age.

Whether or not there is an increased risk of thromboembolism and of endometrial or mammary cancer in predisposed persons with time is a debatable point, and further investigations are needed in order to clarify this matter. An important finding is that the benefits of a prophylactic treatment are very rapidly lost when the medication is withdrawn; osteoporosis, for instance, can develop very quickly once oestrogen therapy is discontinued in the post-menopause and speedily progress to the levels found in untreated people (Lindsay et al., 1976).

## PROPHYLACTIC OESTROGEN MEDICATION

There is sound evidence of a prophylactic effect of oestrogens against post-menopausal osteoporosis, and against atrophic changes in the urogenital target organs. Oestrogens may also have some effect against the deterioration of psychic functions which usually occurs in old age, and against skin atrophy. It is felt that methods are urgently needed in order to predict which patients are likely to develop osteoporosis and fractures in the late post-menopause and which are not, and there are indications that such methods will be known in the near future. A prophylactic effect against athero-sclerosis has not so far been shown, but it seems that oestrogens, certainly when given in low therapeutic doses, do not have a deleterious effect on vascular diseases.

## CONTRAINDICATIONS

There is some difference of opinion as to whether or not the contra-indications for oral hormone contraceptives should indiscriminately be taken to apply also to low-dose oestrogen therapy used for the treatment of climacteric complaints. It is generally agreed, however, that the main contraindications – thromboembolism, myocardial infarction, and cerebrovascular diseases – should, until there is evidence to the contrary, be regarded as applying in both instances.

Regarding cancer, a history of cervical cancer is not a contra-indication for oestrogen therapy, but critical reservation is necessary where endometrial cancer is concerned. There is, however, no indication that oestrogen therapy will adversely influence the cure rate of Stage I or II endometrial cancer patients who have earlier been satisfactorily operated upon or who have undergone radiation therapy (see also Burch et al., 1975). If there is any doubt, nortestosterones or androgens should be given.

For cases of advanced mammary cancer there is a well-approved scheme of oestrogen combined with an androgen or progestogen. High doses of oestriol have also been given with promising results of remission and clinical improvement (Lemon). As far as peri-menopausal women with early stages of breast cancer are concerned, several participants at the workshop referred to patients whose climacteric complaints had been treated with oestrogens after a specific breast cancer therapy. No negative effects of oestrogen medication had been seen in these cases with respect to the further course of the disease. Because of the apparent breast cancer inhibiting properties of oestriol in animal experiments (Lemon, 1978), the administration of oestriol is recommended in selected post-mammary cancer patients. Progestogens may also be given. Receptor studies have so far not been helpful regarding the choice of hormone therapy in post-cancer cases with climacteric complaints.

## RISK FACTORS

Much has been written in recent years concerning the increased risk of various different diseases occurring when women are given oestrogen therapy. Most of this has been based on the theory that the complications which can be expected to arise when women are given oestrogens in the peri- and post-menopause are the same as those seen in certain women taking oestrogens in oral contraceptives.

This theory is now being questioned. Recent results indicate that treatment with natural oestrogens in low doses has no significant effects on glucose metabolism, on lipids, or on liver enzymes (Studd and McKay Hart). Further, some of the changes which do occur after therapy is begun have been found to disappear after some time even though the therapy is continued, and most changes which occur disappear once the medication is withdrawn.

Nevertheless, the concept that certain risk factors do exist for women being treated with oestrogens in the peri- and post-menopause (Lauritzen, 1978) is widely accepted. It is felt, however, that when these risks are taken into account when therapy is being prescribed, the likelihood of such complications actually developing is reduced. No proof of this supposition exists at the present time, however, and it is a fact that complications sometimes arise in women in whom no risk factors are apparent.

Risk factors for thromboembolism, diabetes, gallbladder diseases, and for mammary and endometrial cancer should certainly be respected. These include a familial-genetic predisposition, obesity, old age, hyperlipidaemia, and hypertension. In addition, it has been shown conclusively that the most important risk factor for vascular complications is smoking, and some discussants at this meeting went so far as to formulate that women over 40 should either smoke and not take oestrogens, or take oestrogens and refrain from smoking.

## GENERALIZATIONS ABOUT OESTROGENS

It is sometimes said, even by so-called experts, that oestrogens *cause*, for instance, coagulation changes, thrombosis, and cancer. It must

127

be stressed that such generalizations are quite uncritical and un-justified. Different oestrogens have different ranges of effects and side-effects, and both effects and side-effects are strictly dose-dependent. Therefore, when a statement concerning the effects or side-effects of 'oestrogens' is made the oestrogen being referred to should be stated, and so should the dose level involved. The duration of the treatment and pertinent risk factors in the patient or in the population should also be mentioned.

## INFORMING THE PATIENT

Nowadays most women are aware of the existence of oestrogen therapy before coming for treatment for menopausal complaints, but they are often badly informed about it, and are sometimes in a state of anxiety.

When talking to his patient the prescribing physician should allude to the risks as well as to the benefits of the therapy, but in such a way as to avoid creating fear. He should stress the point that in the absence of any contraindications, oestrogen therapy, properly individualized and supervised by him, will be very safe and that the patient will receive all the benefits of the hormonal therapy whilst avoiding any possible risks (Haspels). The co-operation of the patient is an important aspect of successful oestrogen therapy. Regular check-ups whilst on oestrogen therapy bring the added advantage of the early detection of symptoms and diseases, whether they are related to the administration of oestrogens or not. If co-operation is not guaranteed, and if the patient is against an oestrogen treatment, strong attempts should not be made to persuade her to proceed with it.

## MINIMAL REQUIREMENTS OF CONTROL IN OESTROGEN THERAPY

The minimal requirements for control in oestrogen therapy are a careful anamnesis and a thorough physical examination to ensure that there are no contraindications, to identify the pertinent risk factors, and to select the best treatment for the individual patient. A gynaecological examination, including the taking of a vaginal smear, and an examination of the breasts are necessary. The blood pressure should be measured and urinary glucose should be checked. A measurement of liver enzymes is only necessary if there is a cause for concern because of the patient's history or symptoms. These routine investigations should be repeated every 6 months. It was postulated that, ideally, an aspiration curettage and a mammogram should be performed before treatment is begun and periodically thereafter (Haspels). It was felt, however, that this would be impossible in general practice, primarily because of the cost factor, and that such checks have to be restricted to risk patients.

## ENDOMETRIAL AND MAMMARY CANCER

Since 1976 (Lauritzen, 1976) several aspects of the relationship between oestrogens and cancer have become more clear. It seems to be true that oestrogens in themselves are not carcinogenic, but that they may be facultatively co-carcinogenic in some instances. Special conditions are required in order for cancer to arise and develop; these include a familial-genetic predisposition, influence of real carcinogenics, DNS repair defects, immuno defects, ionizing radiation, ontogenetic malformation of the target organs, local chronic regenerative irritation, old age, metabolic diseases, prolonged unopposed influence of growth promoting agents (like oestrogens), and the lack of antagonistic hormones (like progestogens). Some statistics point to the possibility that the co-carcinogenicity of oestrogens may be diminished by low doses, cyclical administration, and the addition of a sufficient dose of a progestogen. In this case the progestogen should be added for 10 days each month in a dose sufficiently high to cause secretory transformation and a complete shedding of the endometrium upon withdrawal.

## THERE IS NO INDICATION THAT OESTRONE IS MORE CARCINOGENIC THAN OESTRADIOL

Several retrospective studies and one prospective one have recently been carried out in the eastern United States and in Europe in which a correlation between previous oestrogen intake and the occurrence of cancer did not emerge (Nachtigall *et al.*, 1976; Uyttenbroeck and Wauters, 1976; Horwitz and Feinstein, 1977; Lauritzen *et al.*, 1977; Pfleiderer, 1977; Rauramo, 1977). This finding is strangely different from that of several studies conducted specifically in the western United States (Smith *et al.*, 1975; Ziel and Finkle, 1975; Mack *et al.*, 1976; Gray *et al.*, 1977). The difference is, perhaps, to be explained by the fact that in some parts of the United States, at least in the past, rather high doses of oestrogens have been administered on a continuous basis, and progestogens have not always been added.

## COST/BENEFIT AND RISK/BENEFIT RATIOS

An attempt has been made to establish the cost/benefit ratio of oestrogen therapy around the time of the menopause and in the post-menopause (Utian, 1978). It is, of course, difficult to quantify all the variables, and some are not measurable at all. It must be said, however, that the cost of oestrogen therapy is relatively low. Oestrogen therapy and the resultant medical prophylactic supervision *per se* may seem to increase the likelihood of a women being operated upon or having to be treated with additional medicaments. However, the prophylactic effects of oestrogen medication on osteoporosis, bone fractures, and their sequelae, is thought to have a cost-saving effect, and this alone is considered enough to make the cost/benefit ratio positive. The same is probably true for the risk/benefit ratio.

The evidence available at the present time suggests that there is no significant increase of morbidity or mortality for oestrogen users, but rather a slight decrease, and it may be that this is attributable to the strict supervision of the patient which, involving regular medical check-ups, results in the early detection of adverse physical developments not all of which are connected with the administration of the oestrogens (Burch *et al.*, 1975).

## RESEARCH NEEDS

The participants in this workshop considered the following research needs still to apply:

(1) There is need to develop new effective oestrogen preparations which would have a more ideal range of desired effects than the present preparations without undesired side-effects. The ideal oestrogen would not stimulate the endometrium, but

would have a good proliferative and trophic effect on the vaginal wall, the urethra, and the bladder. It would moderately decrease $\beta$-lipoprotein cholesterol, and increase phospholipids, but not triglycerides. It would not exert cholestatic activity, influence coagulation factors, alter glucose metabolism, or increase blood pressure or body weight. It would, however, have strong calcium-retaining and good anti-osteoporotic effects.

(2) Convenient and effective ways of administering oestrogens are sought, other than oral, intramuscular, and via implantations. The aim would be to achieve more physiological blood plasma levels, and a reduction in the incidence and number of side-effects.

(3) Simple, but efficient, screening methods are required in order to detect which patients would be at risk for severe side-effects or other complications whilst under oestrogen therapy.

(4) Similarly, a screening method, or, at least, early diagnostic tools, are needed in order to know which patients are likely to develop osteoporosis and bone fractures in later life if untreated.

(5) More needs to be known about anticarcinogenic hormonal manipulation.

(6) Sensible guide-lines regarding therapy should be established for the prescribing physician; these would probably include advice to use the lowest possible dose, to administer the oestrogens cyclically, to add a progestogen for 10 days each month, and to conduct medical check-ups twice a year.

(7) Prospective studies are needed on the risks which may occur during oestrogen therapy, and research needs to be undertaken in order to find ways of preventing these materializing.

(8) Prospective studies are also needed in order to identify and to quantify the benefits of oestrogen therapy.

# References

Burch, J. C., Byrd, B. F. and Vaughn, W. K. (1975). The effects of long-term estrogen administration to women following hysterectomy. In: *Estrogens in the Post-menopause* (P. A. van Keep and C. Lauritzen, eds.), Front. Hormone Res., **3**, pp. 208–214. (Basel: Karger)

Gray, L. A., Christopherson, W. M. and Hoover, R. N. (1977). Estrogens and endometrial cancer. *Obstet. Gynecol.*, **49**, 385

Horwitz, R. I. and Feinstein, A. R. (1977). New methods of sampling and analysis to remove bias in case-control research: no association found for estrogens and endometrial cancer. *Clin. Res.*, **25**, 459

Lauritzen, C. (1976). Oestrogens and endometrial cancer. In: *Clinics in Obstetrics and Gynaecology* (R. B. Greenblatt and J. W. W. Studd, eds.), Vol. 4, pp. 145–167. (London: W. B. Saunders)

Lauritzen, C. (1978). Management of the patient at risk. In: *Estrogen Therapy – The Benefits and Risks* (C. Lauritzen and P. A. van Keep, eds.), Front. Hormone Res., Vol. 5, pp. 230–247. (Basel: Karger)

Lauritzen, C., Wolf, A. S. and Strabl, M. (1977). A retrospective study concerning postmenopausal estrogen therapy and endometrial cancer. In: *Proceedings of the Second International Meeting on Endometrial Cancer and Related Topics* (M. J. Brush, R. W. Taylor and R. J. King, eds.). (London: Ballière Tindall)

Lemon, H. M. (1978). Clinical and experimental aspects of the anti-mammary carcinogenic activity of estriol. In: *Estrogen Therapy – The Benefits and Risks* (C. Lauritzen and P. A. van Keep, eds.), Front. Hormone Res., Vol. 5, pp. 155–173. (Basel: Karger)

Lindsay, R., Hart, D. M., Aitken, J. M., McDonald, E. B., Anderson, J. B. and Clarke, A. (1976). Long-term prevention of post-menopausal osteoporosis by oestrogen. *Lancet*, **i**, 1038

Mack, T. M., Pike, M. C., Henderson, B. E., Pfeffer, R. J., Gerkins, V. R., Arthur, M. and Brown, S. E. (1976). Estrogens and endometrial cancer in a retirement community. *N. Engl. J. Med.*, **294**, 1262

Nachtigall, L., Nachtigall, R. M., Nachtigall, R. B. and Beckman, E. M. (1976). Oestrogens and endometrial carcinoma. *N. Engl. J. Med.*, **294**, 848

Pfleiderer, A. (1977). Risk factors for endometrial cancer. In: *Proceedings of the Second International Meeting on Endometrial Cancer and Related Topics* (M. J. Brush, R. W. Taylor and R. J. King, eds.). (London: Ballière Tindall)

Rauramo, L. (1977). Oestrogen therapy and endometrial cancer. In: *Proceedings of the Second International Meeting on Endometrial Cancer and Related Topics* (M. J. Brush, R. W. Taylor and R. J. King, eds.). (London: Ballière Tindall)

Smith, D. C., Prentice, R., Thompson, D. J. and Hermann, W. L. (1975). Association of exogenous estrogens and endometrial carcinoma. *N. Engl. J. Med.*, **293**, 1164

Utian, W. H. (1978). Application of cost-effectiveness analysis to post-menopausal estrogen therapy. In: *Estrogen Therapy – The Benefits and Risks* (C. Lauritzen and P. A. van Keep, eds.), Front Hormone Res., Vol. 5, pp. 26–40. (Basel: Karger)

Uyttenbroeck, F. and Wauters, ?. ?. (1976). L'influence des contraceptives oraux, des progestogènes et des oestrogènes dans la genèse des lésions precancéreuses et cancéreuses de l'appareil genital et du skin. Presented before the *Soc. Belge-Pays-Bas d'Obstét. et Gynéc.* Antwerp

Ziel, H. K. and Finkle, W. D. (1975). Increased risk of endometrial carcinoma among users of conjugated estrogens. *N. Engl. J. Med.*, **293**, 1167

# The male climacteric

## Moderator: E. Nieschlag

Department of Experimental Endocrinology, Universitäts-Frauenklinik, Munich, West Germany

*Participants invited to present their views at this workshop included:*

O. Benkert (West Germany)
F. Comhaire (Belgium)
P. Doerr (West Germany)
H. Schmidt (West Germany)
M. Serio (Italy)

This workshop concentrated on the physiology of testicular function in advancing age, on clinical symptoms and possible syndromes in men during advancing age, on correlations between the endocrinological findings and the symptoms, and finally on therapeutic aspects.

## PHYSIOLOGY OF TESTICULAR FUNCTION IN RELATION TO AGE

The plasma testosterone concentrations in men throughout life from conception to senescence show a characteristic pattern. A first peak occurs during weeks 14 to 16 of fetal life at the time of sexual differentiation. A second peak is encountered shortly after birth followed by a phase of relative quiescence up to the age of puberty when a sharp increase in plasma testosterone occurs. The concentrations achieved at the end of puberty, are maintained up to the age of about 50 years. From the sixth decade onwards a slow decrease in plasma testosterone occurs.

The decrease occurring with increasing age has been documented in several studies (Vermeulen *et al.*, 1972; Nieschlag *et al.*, 1973; Pirke and Doerr, 1973). Investigations of the bound and free fraction of circulating plasma testosterone have revealed that the binding increases with advancing age. Thus, the biologically active free plasma testosterone fraction decreases even more than the measurement of total plasma testosterone would suggest (Pirke and Doerr, 1975). Further, the concentrations of testosterone and its precursors in testicular venous blood decrease with age (Serio *et al.*, 1977), indicating a decrease in the testicular testosterone production. Exact measurements have shown that the testosterone blood production rates are lower in older men and the metabolic clearance rate also decreases slightly. These two factors result in a more pronounced fall in urinary testosterone excretion (Schmidt, 1968) than in plasma testosterone concentrations.

Simultaneous with the decrease in plasma testosterone an increase in plasma oestradiol occurs in the total as well as in the free fraction of the steroid (Pirke and Doerr, 1973; Kley *et al.*, 1974; Rubens *et al.*, 1974). This increase in oestrogens is quite in contrast to the decrease seen in menopausal women. The increased oestradiol concentrations may be responsible for an only moderate increase in LH and FSH concentrations in men as compared to the steep increase in gonadotrophins in females during climacterium and post-climacterium.

In men there is not only a decrease in Leydig cell function but also a reduction in the adrenal androgens and androgen precursor secretion. This decrease is most pronounced for DHA and DHA sulphate (Comhaire). However, the glucocorticoid production hardly changes with advancing age. This was interpreted as a shift from the androgen production required for reproductive functions to the more vital production of glucocorticoids.

HCG-stimulation tests have shown that the endocrine capacity of the testes decreases with advancing age (Nieschlag *et al.*, 1973). While the response to a standardized HCG-stimulation with 5000 U/daily for 3 days resulted in a 2.0- to 2.5-fold increase of plasma testosterone in younger men, this response decreased dramatically from the sixth decade onwards so that finally no response could be measured in senescence. The pituitary function does not show any age-related changes as demonstrated by the increase in plasma gonadotrophins with decreasing androgen concentrations and by an unaltered response to LH-RH in older compared to younger men. These results clearly point to the testes as the primary cause of the decreasing testicular function in age. Thus, a type of primary hypogonadism occurs. Most likely these alterations are due to changes in blood flow through the testes. However, to date no exact measurements of testicular blood flow have been performed in men, but histology of the testes showed sclerosis of the arteries.

On histological examination, Tillinger (1957) found a decrease in the number of Leydig cells per tubule with advancing age. However, other investigators have found different results and even Leydig cell hyperplasia was observed (Kothari and Gupta, 1974). The investigations are mainly based on autopsy material and are thus not representative of the normal population. Although difficult to perform in healthy men, the histological investigations seem to require re-evaluation.

Only scanty data on the various ejaculate parameters are available from older men. It appears that the sperm counts are unaltered. However, when taking the prolonged abstinence into account, spermatogenesis seems to be decelerating. Sperm motility also appears to be decreasing. Certain biochemical constituents of the seminal plasma such as fructose show an age-dependent decrease.

Thus, the involution of testicular functions with advancing age is well established. However, this is a slow process starting during the sixth decade of life and slowly progressing during senescence. Hence, a comparison with the relatively abrupt female climacteric is not warranted.

## CLINICAL SYMPTOMS

Various clinical symptoms encountered in men with advancing age have been associated with the declining endocrine function of the testes. Some older men complain of decreasing potency and libido. Some complain about fatigability, decreasing productivity and concentration, depressions, anxiety and sleep disturbances, hot flushes, sweating, tachycardia and skin-atrophy. These symptoms occurring randomly in patients in advancing age led to the coining of the term 'male climacteric syndrome' during the 1930s, assuming an endocrine origin as in women (Werner, 1939). However, are we really justified in talking of about a 'male climacteric syndrome'?

In fact, this syndrome does not exist in psychopathological terms, nor has it been described satisfactorily as a pathological entity. Only single symptoms exist, such as depression and impotence, and they should be considered as such and not as part of a syndrome (Benkert). Approximately 10 000 male out-patients claiming to be suffering from the male climacteric have been evaluated statistically. No age-related increase in the frequency of depression, fatigability and decreased activity was found. There was, however, an age-related increase in sexual disturbances, insomnia, diminished memory functions. These alterations occurred slowly over a long period and there was no sudden change during a distinct phase of life. In order to reveal combinations of symptoms an analysis of configuration frequency was carried out for 12 symptoms in nearly 5000 male patients aged 45–65 years. There were only three combinations of two related symptoms occurring with a higher than expected frequency: sexual disturbances and sweating, sexual disturbances and nervousness, constipation and insomnia (Kies, 1974).

In conclusion, there is an increasing incidence of certain symptoms with advancing age, especially sexual disturbances, memory dysfunction and insomnia. However, the syndrome 'male climacteric' does not exist as a pathological entity and we are only justified to identify, diagnose and treat those symptoms.

Since there are no menses and hence no cessation of menses in men the term 'male menopause' is a nonsensical one which should be avoided.

## CORRELATION BETWEEN ENDOCRINOLOGICAL FINDINGS AND CLINICAL SYMPTOMS

Although the term 'male climacteric' has been used for four decades and more sophisticated methods for the evaluation of testicular function have become available, there has been little attempt to correlate the clinical symptoms with the endocrinological findings. Two recently performed studies were presented at this workshop. Schmidt investigated 78 patients complaining of the symptoms described above. The basal plasma testosterone values in these patients were not different from an age-matched control group. A short-term intravenous HCG-test did not reveal any differences between these groups. The patients were subjected to a battery of psychometric tests and no correlation between the testosterone concentrations and the results of these tests was found. Benkert performed a carefully controlled study in men complaining predominantly of sexual impotence (disturbed erection existing for 1 year, organic causes excluded, acute partner problems absent). There were no differences in the endocrinological findings in the group of patients aged 45 to 60 years and the group aged 61 to 74 years nor was there a difference compared to healthy men.

These two studies were considered as indicating the lack of correlation between endocrinological findings and clinical symptoms. However, it was felt that more thorough studies, including a wider range of parameters, are required before final conclusions can be reached.

## THERAPEUTIC ASPECTS

The male climacteric cannot be considered as a psychopathological entity and a correlation between the symptoms of advancing age and endocrinological findings has not been established. Nevertheless, testosterone has been used for the treatment of these symptoms ever since it became available for therapeutic purposes. Injectable testosterone esters (testosterone propionate and oenanthate) and more recently synthetic androgens have mainly been used. There were, however, only occasional reports on the effectiveness of these preparations, usually indicating positive results.

Schmidt, in the first well-controlled study mentioned above, applied 75 mg mesterolone daily over a period of 5 weeks. A placebo group was included. There was no significant difference between the placebo and the mesterolone groups concerning the psycho-vegetative symptoms, activity and performance, or mood and feelings. The mesterolone-treated patients showed a tendency for improved sexual functions and a significant effect on personality factors, such as emotional lability and masculine self-image, was found. During the discussion it was pointed out that 75 mg mesterolone is not a full replacement dose. It is questionable whether mesterolone can be used for a full testicular substitution therapy; at least 150 mg would be required for that purpose.

In another well-controlled study Benkert treated patients with disturbed potency in advancing age. Sixteen men received the orally effective testosterone undecanoate and 20 received placebo for 8 weeks. Both groups showed significant improvement, yet there was no difference between the androgen treated and placebo treated groups.

Thus, no convincing evidence for the therapeutic effectiveness of androgens in the treatment of age-related symptoms has been produced to date. More controlled studies are required which should also include the 'classical' injectable testosterone esters. There is as yet no firm basis to advise for or against the use of androgens in patients complaining of the symptoms of increasing age. However, when administering androgens certain guide-lines should be followed. As androgens may not induce prostatic carcinoma but will further its growth, the prostate should be regularly investigated in patients receiving androgens. Biochemical parameters such as the radio-immunoassay for acid phosphatase may prove to be of value when monitoring prostatic function. $17\alpha$-alkylated androgens such as $17\alpha$-methyl-testosterone, known to cause liver function disturbances (cholostasis, peliosis and subnormal scintigraphic liver scans), should not be administered.

## References

Kies, N. (1974). Die klimakterische Symptomatologie aus klinisch-psychologischer Sicht. *Med. Welt.*, **25,** 228

Kley, H. K., Nieschlag, E., Bidlingmaier, F. and Krüskemper, H. L. (1974). Possible age-dependent influence of estrogens on the binding of testosterone in plasma of adult men. *Horm. Metab. Res.*, **6**, 213

Kothari, L. K. and Gupta, A. S. (1974). Effect of ageing on the volume, structure and total Leydig cell content of the human testis. *Int. J. Fertil.*, **19**, 140

Nieschlag, E., Kley, H. K., Wiegelmann, W., Solbach, H. G. and Krüskemper, H. L. (1973). Lebensalter und endokrine Funktion der Testes des erwachsenen Mannes. *Dtsch. Med. Wochenschr.*, **98**, 1281

Pirke, K. M. and Doerr, P. (1973). Age related changes and interrelationships between plasma testosterone, oestradiol and testosterone-binding globulin in normal adult males. *Acta Endocrinol. (Kbh.)*, **74**, 792

Pirke, K. M. and Doerr, P. (1975). Age related changes in free plasma testosterone, dihydrotestosterone and oestradiol. *Acta Endocrinol. (Kbh.)*, **80**, 1971

Rubens, R., Dhont, M. and Vermeulen, A. (1974). Further studies on Leydig cell function in old age. *J. Clin. Endocrinol.*, **39**, 40

Schmidt, H. (1968). Testosteronausscheidung bei männlichen Personen unter normalen und pathologischen Bedingungen. *Acta Endocrinol. (Kbh.)*, Suppl. 128

Serio, M., Cattaneo, S., Borrelli, D., Gonnelli, P., Pazzagli, M., Forti, G., Fiorelli, G., Giannotti, P. and Giusti, G. (1977). Age-related changes in androgenic hormones in human spermatic venous blood. In: *Androgens and Antiandrogens* (L. Martini and M. Motta, eds.). (New York: Raven Press)

Tillinger, K. G. (1957). Testicular morphology. *Acta Endocrinol. (Kbh.)*, Suppl. 30

Vermeulen, A., Rubens, R. and Verdonck, L. (1972). Testosterone secretion and metabolism in male senescence. *J. Clin. Endocrinol.*, **34**, 730

Werner, A. A. (1939). The male climacteric. *J. Am. Med. Assoc.*, **112**, 1441

# Other communications

*The following papers were presented during the 'free communication' sessions. The addresses of the first-named authors are included in the list of contributing participants which begins on page ix.*

## I – SOCIAL, CULTURAL, EPIDEMIOLOGICAL, AND RELATED ASPECTS

La ménopausie – the birth of a syndrome – *J. Wilbush (Canada)*

Is the menopausal age rapidly changing? – *C. Bengtsson, O. Lindquist and L. Redvall (Sweden)*

The effect of smoking on menopausal age – *O. Lindquist and C. Bengtsson (Sweden)*

Menopausal effects on risk factors for ischaemic heart disease – *C. Bengtsson and O. Lindquist (Sweden)*

The effect of menopausal age on osteoporosis – *O. Lindquist, C. Bengtsson, T. Hansson and B. Roos (Sweden)*

The clinical features of the onset of menopause and its relation to the length of pregnancies and lactation – *M. L. Batrinos, C. Panitsa-Faflia, S. Pitoulis, S. Pavlou, G. Piaditis, T. Alexandridis and C. Liappi (Greece)*

An attempted differentiation of psychocultural from somato-physiological factors in the menopausal syndrome by the use of ERT – *E. S. Kohane, T. Nathan and M. Gardos (Israel)*

Carbohydrate metabolism in normal healthy and potentially diabetic post-climacteric women – *J. A. Goldman (Israel)*

## II – ASPECTS OF THERAPY

The effect of oestriol on plastic vaginal surgery in post-menopausal women – *S. J. Mantalenakis, G. Eleutheriadis, D. Kesidis and P. Tampakoudis (Greece)*

Effect of oestriol succinate on clear urine cystopathy – *V. Zaragoza Orts, J. Zaragoza Orts, J. Gambini Ricapa and P. Olivas (Spain)*

Five years' evaluation of natural oestrogens in menopausal complaints – *A. M. C. M. Schellen and J. H. Branolte (The Netherlands)*

The treatment of post-menopausal syndrome by monthly oral doses of quinestrol – *S. Anderman, O. E. Jaschevatzky, A. Shalit and S. Grünstein (Israel)*

Serum FSH, LH, and PRL levels in post-menopausal women on cyclofenil treatment – *T. Nencioni, A. Miragoli, F. Dorato, M. G. Bertaglia and C. Antolini (Italy)*

A study of hormone replacement therapy at the menopause – *L. Dennerstein and G. D. Burrows (Australia)*

The treatment of menopausal symptoms with oral oestrogens and the pre- and post-treatment oestradiol FSH and LH levels – *Z. Durmus, O. Iskit and G. Güven (Turkey)*

Effects of sex steroids on lipid levels – *R. Borenstein, N. L. Stahl and R. B. Greenblatt (USA)*

Recovery of clotting factors subsequent to oestrogen medication – *E. S. Kohane and B. Hochstädt (Israel)*

The effects of long-term therapy with oestriol succinate on the haemostatic mechanism in post-menopausal women – *J. L. Toy, J. A. Davies and G. P. McNicol (United Kingdom)*

The lipid theory of atherosclerosis: beneficial effect of pure sex hormones on lipidogram – *M. Oettinger, J. Shani, M. Sharf, N. Naveh, G. Brook, M. Aviram and G. Dankner (Israel)*

Gonadotrophin release in post-menopausal women receiving graded sequential oestrogen-progestogen therapy – *D. W. Sturdee (United Kingdom)*

Treatment of post-menopausal syndrome with oestriol: clinical and laboratory investigations – *D. Kaskarelis, P. Calfopoulos, D. Lolis and D. Aravantinos (Greece)*

Plasma concentrations of oestrone, oestradiol-17$\beta$, oestriol, and gonadotrophins following application of various oestrogen preparations after oophorectomy and in the natural menopause – *J. R. Strecker, C. Lauritzen and L. Goessens (West Germany)*

The effects of oestrogen therapy in peri-menopausal women on transcortin – *U. Schwartz, R. Volger, L. Moltz and J. Hammerstein (West Germany)*

Plasma testosterone and psychotropic effects of an oral androgen in ageing men with psycho-vegetative symptoms – *H. Schmidt, E. Kaiser, N. Kies and G. Maas (West Germany)*

## III – ENDOCRINE ASPECTS

Pituitary hormonal profile in menopause – *M. L. Batrinos, C. Panitsa-Faflia, S. Pitoulis, S. Pavlou, G. Piaditis and T. Alexandridis (Greece)*

Analysis of serum concentrations of oestradiol, luteinizing hormone, and follicle-stimulating hormone during menstrual cycles in peri-menopausal women – *T. Abe, Y. Yamaya, Y. Wada, K. Takahashi and M. Suzuki (Japan)*

A comparison of the effects of physiological and psychological stresses on post-menopausal endogenous oestrogen levels – *S. Ballinger and J. Krivanek (Australia)*

The combines LH-RH + TRH test in post-menopausal patients. 'Preferential LH response': an index of previous oestrogenicity? – *S. Geller and R. Scholler (France)*

Leukocyte alkaline phosphatase (LAP) activity in post-menopausal women and its hormonal regulation – *Y. Z. Diamant, H. Zuckerman and W. Z. Polishuk (Israel)*

Influence of oestrogen therapy on hidroxyiprolinuria during the menopause – *L. Schubert (Italy)*

The fate of a large bolus of exogenous oestrogens administered in menopausal women – *M. F. Aksu, V. A. Tzingounis and R. B. Greenblatt (USA)*

Age dependent hormonal changes in the human male – *H. Sköldefors, K. Carlstrom, P. Eneroth and M. Furuhjelm (Sweden)*

## IV – VAGINAL CYTOLOGY

Cytologic evaluation of hormonal dynamic in the post-menopause – *A. Schachter, A. Segall and E. Avram (Israel)*

The incidence of atrophic smears in 1000 unselected post-menopausal women and in 200 menopausal patients with genital cancer – *M. Eustratiades, E. Tamvakopoulou, C. Panitsa-Faflia, B. Papatheodorou and M. L. Batrinos (Greece)*

Oestrogen treatment of the post-menopause: a cytologic assessment – *J. Hustin (Belgium)*

# V – THE ENDOMETRIUM

Serum levels of total dehydroepiandrosterone and total oestrone in post-menopausal women with and without endometrial cancer – *M. Furuhjelm, K. Carlstrom, M. G. Damber, I. Joelsson, N. O. Lunell and B. von Schoultz (Sweden)*

Steroidogenesis in post-menopausal women with endometrial carcinoma – *J. G. Schenker, B. Eckstein and E. Okun (Israel)*

The role of DHEA and DHEAS as pre-hormones in post-menopausal women – *J. H. H. Thijssen, R. Andriesse and J. Poortman (The Netherlands)*

Endometrium in the post-menopause – *M. J. Casey, T. J. Madden, E. McLucas and A. W. Kennedy (USA)*

Post-menopausal bleeding – *S. J. Joel-Cohen, Y. Ovadia and H. Levavi (Israel)*

The spectrum of lesions associated with post-menopausal bleeding in Turkey – *C. Babuna and A. Turfanda (Turkey)*

Management of post-menopausal bleeding – *R. D. Gambrell (USA)*

The activity of oestrone at the cellular level in target tissues of post-menopausal women – *M. A. H. M. Wiegerinck, J. Poortman and J. H. H. Thijssen (The Netherlands)*

Determination of sexual steroids in serum, human myo- and endometrium in correlation to the content of steroid receptors and $17\beta$-hydroxysteroid dehydrogenase activity during different female reproductive stages – *J. Nevinny-Stickel, J. Eiletz, M. Schmidt-Gollwitzer and K. Pollow (West Germany)*

Prevention of endometrial cancer in post-menopausal women with progestogens – *R. D. Gambrell (USA)*

The risk for endometrial carcinoma due to exogenous oestrogen treatment: a case-control study in a Finnish population – *T. Salmi (Finland)*

A comparison of survival in pre- and post-menopausal patients with endometrial carcinoma – *J. Menczer, M. Modan, D. Ezra and D. M. Serr (Israel)*

143

# Index

144